Vascula   .....lu
Syndrome

The Journey Begins

M J Smith

ISBN-13:978-1-5351-9861-5
ISBN-10:1-5351-9861-3

DEDICATION

This book is dedicated to all those who have lost their lives to Vascular Ehlers-Danlos Syndrome, to all the invisible warriors who continue to fight every day. One day we shall find our cure and the unknown will become the known.

Acknowledgements

I would like to thank my family for always being there and for allowing me to share our story to aid in the awareness of Vascular Ehlers-Danlos Syndrome.

I would also like to thank my loving partner, Rachel, for being by my side and pushing me forward in the publication of this story, and not forgetting spending endless hours trawling through text to make it all possible!

Thanks also goes to Kristi for spending the time to aid in the cover design. And to Kendra for guiding me on the best routes to get published.

And of course, the Griffin family at Annabelle's Challenge. The UK's only charity for Vascular Ehlers-Danlos Syndrome. Spreading awareness and raising funds for the knowledge and treatment of patients diagnosed with Vascular Ehlers-Danlos Syndrome.

Special thanks go to Pink Lily, a light in times of darkness. Without you I might have gotten a little lost!

Introduction

So the past few years have been a little strange. I'm 34 years old and just over a year ago I was diagnosed with a rare genetic condition called Vascular Ehlers-Danlos Syndrome. It is more than likely that you will have never heard of this, I had never heard of it before, and let me tell you most doctors have never heard of it. We are a very rare bunch. There are only around 100 patients officially diagnosed with Vascular Ehlers-Danlos in the UK, but there are thought to possibly be as many as 700 of us. A higher amount, but in the grand scheme of things it's still a little rare. There is no cure. There is a distinct lack of awareness. We walk among you often unseen and unheard, fighting through life on a daily basis.

When I began writing this book I had no intention of doing anything with it. It was my own tool for learning to cope with some of the events that have played out in my life. As time has gone by though, it has become so much more. The more I have come to learn about Vascular Ehlers-Danlos the more I have wanted to try and make a difference. Maybe in some way this will help to get the word out there. Perhaps I can set off little ripples in the waters which will eventually turn to waves. I don't know. All I do know is that I can't stand by and not try. Life is precious, life is short and if I can make a little difference in just one persons life then it has all been worthwhile.

The story I am about to take you on is a little twisty. At times it may seem to make no sense. If truth be told though, Vascular Ehlers-Danlos makes no sense really. I've tried to tell it in a way you will easily understand, whether I have been successful in this, well that's for you to decide. Hopefully you will learn a little more about the syndrome, and hopefully you will grasp some concept of what it's like to have a life altering diagnosis thrown at you. Everything I have written is based on real events, but of course, this is only my story and my life. There are worse cases than myself out there, yet some of the struggles we face are shared by many.

In years to come, hopefully one day we will find our cure, or if not a cure then perhaps a way to live safer lives. Until that time though, the name of Vascular Ehlers-Danlos needs to be shouted out. You have to start somewhere, right? So getting awareness is the way to go. This is just my way of trying to give a little back. So pour yourself a cup of tea or coffee, take a seat, sit back, relax and come on join me on this adventure. I will see you on the other side!

CHAPTER 1
THE JOURNEY BEGINS

I lay there, arms crossed over my chest, an emergency buzzer loosely clasped in my left hand so not to accidentally press it. My body rigid, head braced, facing directly upwards, only looking at the angled mirror directly above my eyes. There's a slight chill being sent up and down my spine from the opening of the thin linen hospital gown that I now wear. With a low pitched buzzing the bed begins to slowly slide into the enclosed tube. As my head enters the tight space a feeling of becoming trapped enters my mind. What was a large empty room, has now become a cold tomb.

Motionless, I lay there, daring not to breathe, surrounded by a smooth white shiny surface just inches from my face curving around my body. As the bed comes to a standstill, all that is left is the sound of my heartbeat thumping in my chest, sounding as if every beat is bouncing off the curved walls of the MRI machine.

My eyes focus on the mirror that's attached to the neck brace, trying to take my mind off the enclosed space. With its slight angle it allows me to see out of the end of the tube. It seems like a great distance away, but beyond the end of the tunnel I can see the back of the room. I know the room is empty, but my eyes focus on a giant single paned window that gives sight to a dark room where the silhouettes of two figures loom. For what feels like an age, I lay there, silent, cold, unable to

1

move. The cables attached to my body rubbing against my skin, annoying me, making me want to adjust them out of the way. Still I resist and stay as rigid as a mouse playing dead. The dark silhouettes are now seated, the faint glow of a computer screen casting eerie shadows over one of them. From the darkness, I see the other place what appear to be headphones over their head.

"Are you okay?" A soft gentle female voice comes out of the headphones that are placed awkwardly over my head.

"I'm .. fine" I reply in a shallow croaked voice, as if speaking will hinder the process. Of course I wasn't fine really, if I was I wouldn't be here!

"We are going to begin now. If at any time you feel uncomfortable then please press the buzzer and we will be right here."

Her voice fills me with a little warmth, as I begin to close my eyes. A few seconds later the noise begins, a large banging sound that fights its way through the headphones, a whirring, a thumping, alternating between sounds, reminding me of how a cassette tape would load in an old Commodore 64. The flashes of light on the screen would seem to change in time with the sound of the game loading. A constant droning, which I now have to listen to for the next forty minutes. In complete stillness, not twitching, not itching, not moving a muscle, the seconds feeling like hours, and then it stops. The beating of my own heart is all that remains.

"Are you still okay?"

"Yeah great" I reply as I slightly move my hand up to my bearded chin to scratch the itch that has just begun to annoy me.

"We are now going to do the second scan. For this you will need to hold your breath and remain completely still when I say, and before it's over we will send the dye through, but I will tell you before this happens."

As the voice rings though my head I clasp the buzzer a little harder in my hand, making sure that it is still there if I need to use it. Once again the banging begins, the deep thud reverberating around the curvature of the internals. A few seconds pass by.

"Now I want you to hold your breath, follow my voice, deep breath in, deep breath out, deep breath in and hold."

As I follow the voice I slowly fill my lungs with as much oxygen as possible, not that I feel like there is a lot to take in inside this mechanical tube. With my lungs filled to capacity, I lay there for what seems like an eternity. I begin to feel like I can't hold it any longer, panic starts to fill my body, wanting to expel the oxygen but knowing that if I do the process has to start all over again. I can feel my body wanting to kick out, but I must stay still.

"And breathe" the voice calls out in my head.

"Thank god for that" I thought to myself, another moment longer and I would have been kicking out.

"In a moment we are going to release the dye for the last scan."

The second the voice stopped the MRI started up again, with its usual thumping and whirring. In my right arm I began to feel a warm tingling sensation as the dye begins to flow into my veins. Flowing up my arm and into my shoulder, I could feel it filling up inside of me, in my neck, into my head, the faint tickly warmth spreading through my body, as it starts to go down towards my groin. For a moment I feel like I'm peeing myself, then it is gone.

"All done."

I let out a sigh of relief as the motorised bed begins to whirr and slowly slips me out of this godforsaken enclosure. It is done!

2

So why would I start my story here when there are so many places to begin. Why not start it with the searing pain in my head, with the loss of vision causing ripples of colours blocking everything in sight, with the feeling of lead weights being strapped to my left leg and arm. Why not start it when I was sat in that room being told my life was about to change, not only mine, but of those closest around me. Or maybe even the time I was told I was lucky to be alive, or even luckier not to have some sort of long term physical damage.

Well, I guess the reason behind this, which you will know if you have been inside an MRI machine, is that it gives a slight portrayal of the feeling of loneliness, helplessness. The feeling of being trapped in this tight cocoon unable to move, shallow breaths you take leading to lack of air in the lungs. Being able to see out the end of the tunnel, but having no way to get out. A complete lack of control of what's happening around you; fear, panic, loneliness. It's times like these that the darkness creeps up on you, the monster inside of your subconscious mind, the anger, the rage, the frustration that creeps up on you without realising, taking control of your body and mind.

Here we are then, sat at my keyboard typing away and trying to tell you a story. My name's Dave. Why Dave? Because that's what I'm going to call myself, Dave! I like the name Dave, it flows out of the mouth nicely, easily, and it's not really a name you forget. You can call me David if you like, but you must agree, Dave is a lot better!

I'm 33 years of age. Well technically I'm 33 years and 8 months old, minus a few days, but that's taking things a little too far.

If you would like to get a picture of I what I look like, well I guess I stand at around 5ft 7 to 5ft 8. A friend of mine once told me that they measure in hands, an interesting concept, I liked this. We even worked out the exact conversion rate into inches of what her hand measurement would be. I could probably work out the exact hand measurement for you now and it would make a great universal measuring tool, but I'm not quite sure the world is ready for this.

Weight wise, the last time I checked I was around 13 stone, how many pounds I haven't got the faintest and I'm not interested. I'm not really one to bother about such things. My eyes are brown, a little on the larger side some may say, as is my nose. Its kind of thin, with a lump on the bridge of it. I suppose you could call it a proud Roman nose, not that I have any links to Roman heritage that I know of. I have the blood of the Irish in my veins. This comes from mothers side, her father was Irish and I like to think that this is where my positive attitude and love of life comes from.

My hairstyle......what hair, I shaved that years ago, all that's left is a couple of millimetres of fluff, receded either side, thinning out on the crown and with a protruding part in the middle, which I'm sure in time when my hair has receded back far enough down the side will turn into some sort of roundabout on the front of my head. Perhaps when that happens a complete head shave will be necessary, or maybe a wig with dreadlocks?

Around my small lips, I have an area of beard growth, a goatee! This I have now had for many years. I did try to shave it off once, but I felt a little naked. Walking around feeling the fresh breeze on my non existent chin must have been like feeling the cold air around your loins as you walk along the beach on a windy day, naked. Not that I have actually done that before. When I sit contemplating important matters, I like to run my hands through it, stroking my chin and feeling its wiry softness!

What else would you like to know? I have small feet. Size 8 to be precise, or if I'm really truthful, then size 7. Since we are being truthful, I have webbed toes, not all of them mind, just the two toes next to my big toe. On my left foot the web goes up three quarters of the way, on my right it goes up half way. My hands are small and dainty, some people would say girl's hands, but no, they are my hands!

Well hopefully that's enough to give you some kind of image as to what I look like. I am sure that in your mind's eye, by the end of this book your imagination will have conjured up some obscure image of myself. I'm quite ordinary really, sure I could of made myself out to be some sort of male Adonis, but in this tale I would like to portray everything in an honest tone.

Up until now my life has been quite normal, there has been nothing that really sets it apart from anyone else's; although it would seem, what is normal for me is not quite as normal as I thought. I've grown up by the sea in Lincolnshire, pretty much a rural farming type of area. Grammar school educated, not that this really means a lot as I never really pushed myself in my schooling years, but I still came out all right. My first job at 16 when I left school, was packing bags at local supermarket with the greatest of uniforms. I used to wear a bright red waistcoat, black trousers, white shirt and a black dickie bow. Oh how dapper did I look! Working there were some of the greatest days of my life, no worries, no responsibilities, going to work, coming home, having fun, drinking plenty!

Of course those days didn't last. We grow up, settle down, get married, have a child, get divorced and then spend the rest of the time drifting in and out of relationships. At least that's how it was for me. Not that I'm complaining, this path has taken me on many adventures and there are some great memories tucked away in there as well as the ones that I'd rather tuck away into a little box in the back of my mind!

3

Here we are now then, in the present day. I'm currently working in the tyre industry as a fitter and a salesman. Over the years I seem have grown a love of all things round and rubber, some kind of weird fetish maybe? I don't know, you can decide on that one! It's not the greatest of jobs and I've tried to move away from it a time or two, in what I shall call my drifting years, the past 10 years I guess. But no, somewhere deep inside I must like it!

I live in a rented flat in a small village. Well when I say small it seems to have expanded quite a lot over the years. New housing estates have gone up on the edge of the village and it has enough people to support 4 public houses, 2 restaurants, 3 small shops, a petrol station and even a butchers and a bakery, so it must be getting on in size now. We even have our own bypass.

Life in general had been pretty good. I didn't have any set in stone plans for the future, but it was moving forward. I was living, going to work, going out and dancing the night away .. and my dancing skills were obviously very good given the practice I'd had over the years. Think of someone flailing their arms around wildly in the air, giving a bit of an Irish jig with the fastest footwork you have ever seen and all this completely out of time to the music. That was a skill that had taken me years to develop, and I was so proud of it.

Yes a regular master of the dance floor, and if a Bon Jovi song should crop up, well you should hear me wail like a screaming banshee to the sounds of "Livin' on a Prayer", most impressive. Awesomeness oozed out of my entire body.

Every other weekend I would have my now 10 year old, son. These are the weekends I would enjoy the most. We didn't always do a lot, sometimes we would go to the cinema, sometimes we would just chill out and play the Xbox. When I say play, I meant he would just slaughter me on any game that he would possess. I guess my gaming skills have slowly faded with age! But every moment I spend with him, I appreciate and love so much more than any other. In a way, although I would love to have him live with me full time, I like the fact that he's not always here, because it makes it extra special when he is here. His name is Gordon by the way. Remember Gordon, it may or may not crop up again!

Without further ado, let's just jump back quickly to August, two years ago....that's August 2012 for anyone who's not really paying attention...you should really pay attention! My mind does tend to veer off on a different course sometimes, but you may miss vital information.

So I'm going to make this as quick and as simple as possible. It was a Thursday. The exact date I do not remember, a lot has happened in the last two years, but yes, I know it was a Thursday. I'd had the week off from work, and I had Gordon with me for the week. This day was pretty much a relaxing day. We had been out the day before, firstly to the cinema, and if I recall correctly it was the final instalment of Harry Potter, oh how I dislike the Harry Potter series, but as with any 8 year old of course he liked it! Before this we had been to have a look around a castle, so that Thursday was just a hang out day. We'd played a little football in my parents back garden, and played a little Xbox. You know, all the normal stuff. Only it turns out it didn't happen to be a normal day.

For a few months previously I had been getting migraines. The type of migraines where, lets say you were reading, like you obviously are now, and as you were reading you would notice that letters would begin to disappear. Not all of them, just one at a time in the s me spot of y ur vision. Sort of like what I did there, if you were paying attention to that line of wording. Then you would notice a kind of small jagged tear that would have blocks of colours. Eventually this tear would begin to fill the whole left hand side of the vision. Just a mass of blocked colours obscuring your sight. This would go on for about 30-40 minutes and what followed was the most painful headache on the right hand side of my head. Like a herd of elephants trampling through a corridor on the right hand side of the brain! Terrible, but just a normal migraine right, an aura migraine I think they may be called.

Anyway these had started at a rate of once a month, then they began to hit me twice a month, which I had been to the doctors about and received medication for, but they didn't stop.

Now on this normal Thursday that turned out to be not so normal, something changed. I was sitting there watching Gordon, playing on the Xbox whilst I was texting on my swanky smart phone. I pulled myself up out of my seat and as I did that I immediately saw stars in my vision, my heart began to race, pounding in my chest, getting faster and faster. I felt a sharp pain shear through the right hand side of my head, deep inside of my brain somewhere like a knife had just ripped straight through my skull and was piercing deep inside of my head. Not wanting to disturb or worry Gordon I began to walk into the kitchen.

Beads of sweat were beginning to form on my

forehead. My left leg turned heavy, like a lead weight had suddenly been strapped to it, and each step became a great effort trying to lift it off the floor. As soon as I managed to lift it, it went back down with a deep thud, as though gravity had just doubled on that side of my body. I felt faint, I felt panic, and I felt pain.

At this point, most people would have probably sought help, but being myself and tending to try and ignore these things, and again not wanting to worry Gordon, I got myself a glass of water and went to lay myself down on the bed. I closed my eyes and tried to ignore the pain, ignore the beads of sweat running down my face, ignore the fast paced pounding of my heart.

As I lay there, things began to settle. The knife was still in my head being twisted, however my heart rate began to slow. The stars in my vision began to subside. The head pain I could deal with, as long as everything else had gone I knew I'd be fine. At least until Gordon went home after the weekend and I could get myself to the doctor without raising too much concern. With just the pain in the head remaining, not as sharp as before, but a dull ache, I carried on.

4

The following Monday came, it couldn't have come soon enough. I was meant to be returning to work from my week off, but since that Thursday the pain in the right side of my head hadn't gone away. It remained with me, beating me down, trying to cripple me and confine me to my bed. I kept fighting it, ignoring it, which may have been the wrong thing to do. As they say though, ignorance is bliss. As well as the pain, the problems with my vision had come everyday, for about 40 minutes at some point on the Friday, the Saturday and the Sunday, my vision would begin to blur out. To have so many migraine attacks in such a short period of time, something obviously wasn't right.

When I awoke on the Monday, there it was, the vision, the blocks of colours dancing around my eyesight, hindering my every movement. I picked up the phone to call the doctors. I had to get an appointment and sort myself out. I try not to go to the doctors often, apart from the previous time this year I had been regarding my migraines, I think it had been a few years since my last visit. I didn't often get sick, I didn't catch many colds, I was what you would call reasonably healthy apart from the odd ailment here and there, and the usual aches and pains at times.

Luckily I managed to get an appointment for around 9:15am. By this time my vision was once again back to its full glory. My arms and legs were functioning as they should; just the pain remained, which I was now becoming very much accustomed to. So I was able to drive myself down to the surgery.

I walked into the surgery. It was busy, there were bodies everywhere, coughing, spluttering, people looking sorry for themselves. Hospitals, doctors, have I told you I hate these places? At the reception desk there was a long line of people, one which I thankfully didn't have to join. No, in front of me they had an automated book in system. Technology, you have to love it, it makes our lives so much easier. Across the room I walked. To my right the seats were full; hopefully I wouldn't have to sit down there, the thought of brushing shoulders with someone coughing their guts up was not one I liked. Entering my details into the system and letting them know that I had arrived, the screen flashed back with *"please take a seat in corridor A."*

Corridor A was much better. A long corridor lined

with a few chairs, numerous rooms off to either side. The décor made it feel homely and warm. Wall paper all the way down either side, a nice warm sunsetty orange, not too dark, not too bright, just right. I liked it! The carpet was nice and soft. It can't have been that old, as if it was I'm sure it would have been threadbare with the amount of people that must surely walk up and down it all day. Large green plants lined the corridor. I'm not sure if they were fake plastic ones, or what variety they were. Personally my knowledge on all things green is seriously lacking. In fact, if I had a cactus, it would probably end up dying from lack of water!

I walked to the bottom of the corridor, past about eight doors, four either side. There at the bottom were three empty chairs and to my surprise they looked like rather comfy padded chairs. I planted myself down on one. It was opposite the door of Dr Haramesh. This was apparently the doctor I had an appointment with. I'd never heard of her, never seen her before. At this point I just needed to see a doctor and any would do.

As soon as I sat down a voice came over the tannoy. Emanating from the speaker on the roof came the soft voice of a young lady.

"David Malarkey for Dr Haramesh please."

That was quick, I thought I would at least be waiting ten minutes. Arising from the comfort of my padded chair I walked towards the door, and before entering I gave a light knock. This was the polite way to go into a doctor's office was it not?

"Come in" came that voice from beyond the door. If someone had coughed then I would have never have heard it.

As I entered the room I saw her sitting there. She looked quite elegant, and around the same age as me. I'm not good with ages; maybe she was perhaps a little younger, I'm not sure. But as soon as my eyes set upon her I knew I was going to like her. I don't know if anyone else is like this, but sometimes I can tell by the look of someone that I know whether I'm going to take to them or not. I know you should never judge a book by it's cover, but I always seem to have a good gut instinct. Rarely is it wrong and I had a feeling I wasn't wrong about her.

"Good morning David, please take a seat." Her soft tone came across to my ears like music.

"What can I do for you today?"

As she said this, she looked straight into my eyes. Now my eyes were very heavy and perhaps bulging a little. They had grown weary from the pain that was inside my head, and from an abundant lack of sleep, so I got the feeling she was picking up on this.

I began to explain the occurrence on the Thursday, running through the events trying not to miss anything out. I went back in time a little to give her a history of how the migraines had progressed. How they had suddenly started up, how they had begun to become more frequent, until that day. I also told her that I had been before to ask about them, and was handed a prescription for aspirin.

Whilst I was describing this to her she looked at me inquisitively, paying great attention to everything I was saying. She was listening to what I had to say. This made me feel at ease. No feeling of awkwardness. I've found over the years that some doctors can feel intimidating, but my gut feeling was right, Dr Haramesh was slightly different.

"Okay, well what we will do is put you on a combination of two tablets. These are tablets that should stop the migraines, I want you to take these for a few days and see how you get on. If the pain gets worse or different then come back or phone up straight way. I'm also going to sign you off work until they get in your system. Either way come back and see me in a week's time."

This seemed like a reasonable answer to me, and worthy of a try. Migraines can do funny things to people and can manifest in many different ways. So all being well this would sort me out and I could get back to living my life as soon as possible! I left the room, still with that pain, but feeling relatively good, and back home I went to begin my course of tablets.

5

So the days were beginning to pass by. I was taking the tablets, which for me was a miracle. Call me strange, I know I am in many ways so it doesn't really bother me, but I've always had problems swallowing tablets. I'm not a tablet person. I tend to find that rather than swallow them, they get stuck in my throat and end up being coughed straight back up. Usually I would give up on them, but this time I knew I had to try. Luckily they were the tiniest of things, so once I got used to it they started going down well. Although I did often find myself at the sink for 10 to 15 minutes at a time with countless attempts at trying to get them down. I even went as far as looking on the internet for advice on the best way to swallow them. You may laugh, but you shouldn't, its psychological don't you know.

By the end of the week, the pain was still there. It had not diminished in the slightest. Constantly drumming away at me, that herd of elephants running backwards and forwards, unrelenting on their journey inside of my head. I was growing tired of it. It hurt. All I wanted to do was sleep but I couldn't sleep. When I could sleep I would wake again within the hour. There was one night I remember quite well. Which night I couldn't tell you exactly, but I was sleeping, quite nicely, until I was woken by my own screams of pain. Call me an idiot for ignoring what was going on, but I was scared. I fear everything hospital wise, everything doctor wise. Over the years I had seen too much pain to want to be pulled into that world. So when I woke like that, the burning pain, the lightning bolts bouncing around inside my skull with the power of 10,000 gigawatts, I tried to ignore it and hope it would calm down. For a few minutes it would attack me, sending shivers throughout my body, my muffled screams held back by the sheets clamped tightly between my teeth. The sweat seeped out of every pore in my body, soaking the bed, my body twisting uncontrollably. It was like some sort of nightmare, and what made it worse was that I couldn't hold it like a wounded arm or leg, it was deep inside me and all I could do was roll around. My mind would repeat over and over again,

"A few minutes. A few minutes, it's gonna stop, it's gonna, a few more minutes.."

I kept that mantra of hope in my head, and eventually the thunderstorm would subside. It would ease off and go back to my herd of elephants. These I could cope with. I had now become accustomed to having them there. I just thanked my lucky stars it stopped so I didn't have to head to the hospital.

Monday came around again, slowly but surely. A week of taking the tablets and nothing had changed. So I made another appointment to go back and see Dr Haramesh. This time I was sure the appointment would flow in a different direction. This time I was certain she was going to try something else.

Upon walking into that room, there she was, sat there in her youthfulness. She did seem a little too young to me to be a doctor. I had never spoken to a doctor younger than myself, and now I was certain that she was quite a lot younger. Maybe I was beginning to get old. There were no crows feet around her eyes, in fact no wrinkles anywhere. Her dark skin was smooth and silky.

"Good morning David, how are you feeling today? How are you getting on with the tablets? You don't look too great."

To my surprise she remembered me. I wasn't expecting that. I know it had only been a week, but surely she had seen that many patients by now she would have forgotten this bulging eyed mess of a man that was before her last week?

"I'm not doing so well. The pain is still there, the vision keeps going." Of course I didn't tell her about the night I woke up writhing around like a lunatic. I had a feeling she wouldn't have been happy with me. I maybe should have, but I didn't want to.

"What I'm going to do then is refer you to a neurologist and send you for an MRI. I will try and get you in as quickly as possible."

With these words, concern began to fill my body. I wanted the pain sorting, but I didn't want anything to be wrong! A fear was beginning to build up inside of me, a fear of my own body and what it was trying to do to me.

There was nothing more to say really. What had to be done was being done. I was now embarking on a journey with so many twists and turns and where it would end up leading me was anybody's guess.

I hoped that everything would be all right. That this would all turn out to be nothing. I had a full life ahead of me yet, a lot to live for and a lot of things I wanted to do. I didn't have time for problems like these. I just wanted to get on and be done with it.

6

Over the course of the few months I had numerous tests done, MRI scans, CT scans and at one point I even had a camera shoved down the back of my throat to check out my heart. This is one test that I wouldn't wish on anybody. I'm going to tell you about this one as my memory serves me quite well.

The appointment had been made for mid afternoon. Around 2 or 3pm; the exact time I'm not sure of. For this I hadn't had to travel far, a 45 minute drive away from where I lived, to the local hospital. When I arrived at the hospital I had to go up quite a few floors. There are nine floors in total in this particular hospital. I don't remember which floor it was, but was perhaps the 5th? On getting to the floor it was more like going onto a ward to visit someone. The hospital was basically a rectangular shaped building, with the lifts situated in the centre of the building. So when you went up and stepped out, you would come out into a foyer at the front. Lifts either side of you, two in front and two behind. Turning to the right there was a big window giving sight out to the land in front of you. Down below you could see the car park, the tiny people, looking rather like ants at this height, scurrying around. Beyond the car park it gave way to fields, hundreds of fields as far as the eye could see, cabbages, sprouts and all things vegetable being grown.

Turning out of the lifts to the left gave access to two corridors, one heading north and one heading south. I'm quite sure that they weren't actually northerly or southerly facing, but it shows they are opposite each other right? Anyway, on this occasion I would be turning left out of the lift and turning left again down the corridor. I don't like hospitals, I never have, they always have that strange smell about them. Microwaved meals, disinfectant. Your footsteps always echo or squeak depending on the footwear you have chosen, and the sound of this bounces off the tall wide corridors. I often wonder if a ninja would be able to navigate these places without making a single sound. Maybe one day I should try this! I obviously neglected to tell you that as well as having dancing skills, I'm also quite a ninja, trained in the Tibetan mountains by the kung fu squirrel master.......but that's a story for another time!

So heading down the corridor with tall walls either side I walk towards the nurses station. The nurses station is located on the middle of the square, two squares make the floor, one to the left, one to the right. As I get closer the right hand side opens out to a waiting room. There aren't many people sat around, more empty plastic blue chairs than there are people. This perhaps would be a good thing, so I wouldn't have to wait too long. As I was feeling pretty agitated at having to have this thing shoved down my throat, getting it over and done with quickly would be very good indeed.

I spoke to the nurse at the nurses station, a rather small looking plump lady. If you have ever seen "Lord of the Rings" she did kind of remind me of the angry dwarf, although I have to say, she didn't come across as angry. She was very abrupt, and I don't think I would have liked to say the wrong thing to her in fear of getting my head bitten off in an instant. After making them aware of my presence of greatness, I was seated in one of those plastic blue chairs, not exactly a seat fit for a king such as myself, but I guess the NHS does have its limits on what it can spend on seating.

For about five minutes I sat staring at the clock up above my head. There was no TV, and the magazines were mostly old issues of "Hello" or "OK". It wouldn't seem very manly of me to pick up one of those and start reading.

It was quiet, apart from the occasional cough and splutter from the old man sitting opposite me, voices were whispers, and every now and then you would hear an awkward conversation flowing through the air, then disappearing again as soon as it had come. Seems it's not just me that isn't too keen on these places!

I watched the second hand on the clock ticking round, counting each beat, 1 1000, 2 1000, 3 1000, 4 1000. I wonder how many other people count like that? I may be wrong but I seem to recall hearing a boy counting like that on the film called "Poltergeist", many many moons ago, but I'm sure he was counting the time between lightning strikes to the rumble of thunder to gauge the distance. That would have been an interesting measurement to take on with the hand theory. On this day I also discovered that in actual fact there were sixty seconds in a minute. Who would have thought that. I even checked it five times. Makes me wonder who decided to make it that way.

After my important discovery about time, I was finally called.

"David Malarky please" came a voice from behind my head.

"That's.....me"

Whilst saying this, I awkwardly twisted my neck around to see where the faceless voice had come from, a young nurse stood before and beckoned me to follow her.

"Would you like to come with me please!"

I span round, stumbling on the chair a little, nerves had obviously started to get the better of me giving me an uncoordinated body. The nurse led me to a room which resembled that of an ordinary ward. Six beds lined the edges of the room, three either side, and they were all empty! I was taken across to the middle bed, where she lay me down and began taking down my particulars.

After a long list of the standard boring questions regarding allergies, previous surgeries etc etc, she closed the curtains around the bed and told me to strip down to just my jeans and handed me one of those lovely faded chequered blue gowns in which I felt a strange excitement at wearing.

The nurse left me after telling me that the doctor would be here to see me in a minute to go through the "procedure". That left me with a feeling of trepidation. "Procedure", did she really have to call it that? Making it sound like I was about to be cut open or something? Not the nicest of thoughts running through my head!

The doctor walked through the double doors with a clipboard in hand, threw back my curtains and immediately burst out into conversation.

"Good afternoon David, I'm Doctor Pheodopolopolis and I will be carrying out your procedure today. Do you know why you are having this done?" his tone assertive.

My reply to this man in his beige corduroy trousers, white shirt and Santa tie was,

"Yes, from what I've been told you need to look at the back of my heart and this is the best way to do it."

"That is correct, but do you know what we are looking for?" His eyes gazed at me inquisitively.

"Erm, well no not really. I know it needs to be done but that is all." Something didn't seem quite right in this conversation.

"Okay, well your notes are still on their way here, so I don't know what we are looking for exactly, so what we will do is just look for the usual."

"What? You're going to stick a camera down my throat, when you don't even know why you're doing it?"

I was a little shocked at the fact that they didn't even have my notes. It was bad enough that they had to do it, but to not know what they were looking for? To have to ask me? I am no doctor, I'm the patient. Surely they should be telling me, and reassuring me?

"It's okay, it's quite a common procedure, you will be fine." Ha ha, of course this statement filled me with great confidence.

The doctor left, and a porter came in to push me around to the "procedure" room. As I was pushed through my mind kept wandering to the fact they didn't know why I was having a camera shoved down my throat. I thought the idea of having it done was bad enough, but with the fact that I had always struggled with the tablet swallowing, the thought of having something like that in my throat wasn't exactly filling me with happy thoughts. A coldness was beginning to sweep through my body. As we went back past the waiting room, past the clock where I discovered there were actually sixty seconds in a minute, and towards another room, I felt fear and panic gripping hold of my mind.

Going through some more double doors we came to another big empty room. In the middle of the room was a computer screen, the monitor for the camera I assumed, and a tray laying next to it. The tray for this moment was empty, but it soon wouldn't be. The doctor that filled me with so much confidence was stood next to the monitor clicking away and cycling through screens. He didn't lift his gaze when I entered the room, just carried on about his business. Around the edge of the room there were cupboards aplenty, god only knows what torturous toys lie behind those cupboard doors. I tried to empty my mind and dare not think about it.

"Hello again David" came that elusive voice from the left hand side of the room. There in the corner stood the nurse who had handed me the fine garments that dangled off my body. She was busy stretching out a pair of blue latex gloves and placing them over her hands.

The porter pushed my bed next to where the monitor

sat in the centre of the room.

"Please lie on your right side" the nurse said to me as she cast her gaze to take mine away from what the doctor was doing.

"What I'm going to do is spray the back of your throat to numb it so you won't feel anything. It may be a little uncomfortable but don't panic."

Hmm don't panic, in other words I'm probably going to panic and not like this one bit.

The nurse put one hand on my shoulder and gave a little stroke with her left hand, in the other she held a small spray, of which I couldn't read what it was, I didn't want to. I kept my eyes transfixed on her eyes, away from the sight of anything that was about to happen.

Raising her right hand and signalling for me to open my mouth, she brought the spray close to me. Two squirts later I felt it hit the back of my throat. A coldness, giving way to a tingly sensation, then nothing, my throat had gone, complete numbness. I tried to swallow, I couldn't swallow. My gaze left her, and I looked to my left where the empty tray was now filled with a gigantic camera, not the small thing I had imagined in my head, but this humongous shaft with a thick girth that was about to be shoved down my throat. My god it was huge. Immense panic now gripped me. This was going to hurt, this wasn't what I imagined. I tried to swallow again, but nothing. I felt like I couldn't breathe, like I had hands clasped around my throat, squeezing so hard, not letting any air in.

"Don't look over there, look at me" she said as she placed her hand on my shoulder again.

It was too late for that, I'd already seen and I was scared. I feared this monstrosity. Every ounce of me wanted to jump up from this bed and run, run until I couldn't run, but I couldn't. I wouldn't have got far, I couldn't even breathe, I couldn't swallow.

My eyes turned and locked onto the deep brown eyes of the nurse, she must have seen the sheer terror in my bulging eyes. I felt her hand come up to me. There was a needle now in her left hand, as soon as I saw that needle it was slyly and quickly jabbed into me. I felt a giant hand grab my head and turn it to the left where the camera lay, only this time the camera wasn't on the tray, it was in the doctors hand, coming up towards me. A mouth guard was immediately placed in my mouth, and saliva was dribbling out because of my inability to swallow. Jesus I was going to drown in my own spit! As soon as the mouth guard was in place, there it was in all its might, surely way too wide to fit down my throat. Flying through the air, straight for the mouth guard. With much precision it slid in and hit the back of my throat, pushed hard and fast, yeah my throat was numb but it hit with such force I thought it was going to break out the back of my neck ... then nothing!

My eyes began to open, heavy, unfocused. I took a small gulp, I say small as my throat was still numb, but not like before, I actually had a throat now. I could feel it slightly, soreness was there. Wondering where the hell I was my eyes started to focus a little more, nothing much to see apart from the curtains that wrapped around my bed. I was back in what I would call the "pre-procedure" room. How I had got there I do not know. The last thing I remember was that gargantuan camera hitting the back of my throat so hard, then nothingness. Like I had just woken up from a dream. If my throat wasn't still slightly numb and sore then I would have thought of it as nothing more than a distant dream.

With that the curtains came back and in walked the doctor again.

"So okay, how do you feel?"

"Fine and dandy" I replied in a weak sarcastic tone, the words slipping away. How would anyone feel after that!

"Well, everything went okay. We didn't find anything so I will write back to your doctor and let him know. A nurse will be along shortly with a cup of tea and a biscuit and then you'll be free to go."

"Gee thanks, that's ace!"

My mind gave a chuckle. Tea and biscuits, is that some sort of prize for letting you have your sadistic way with me and shoving that damn thing down my throat? Thanks doc!

And that was that. A little time passed, I slowly had my cup of tea, swallowing a tiny sip at a time due to the battered and bruised throat that I was now left with. I even managed a few bites of my bland cardboard tasting digestive biscuit. Still, at least the experience was over and I could get out of this place!

CHAPTER 2
THE SEARCH FOR TRUTH

When I started writing this, I did have an aim. But now that aim seems to have gone out of the window. I had a story mapped out in my mind, but I'm no longer following that. We shall save that for another day perhaps. If you bear with me, all will perhaps become clear. I'm now writing from my heart, perhaps not the best of places for things to come from. When you let your heart rule you rather than your head you tend to get burned. Well at least I do anyway. But the heart is a powerful thing, after all it pumps our lifeblood around our bodies and it's what keeps us ticking along all nice and tickety boo!

So after that slight deviation, if you're are keeping up, I was saying that I had been for MRI scans etc etc etc. I had travelled around the country seeing specialist after specialist. Things weren't exactly getting very far though.

The results from some of these various scans showed that:

1. I have had a dissection of the intra-cranial carotid artery.

2. I'd also had a stroke.

I will try not to insult your intelligence here and will not explain what a stroke is, but I will go onto explain what the intra-cranial carotid artery dissection is, as this was the most interesting aspect of what had been found on the MRI scan and as it turns out, quite a rare occurrence.

In layman's terms we have two carotid arteries, one on the left and one on the right. If you feel for the pulse in your neck this is where they reside. Their job is to supply blood to the large front part of the brain, this is where thinking, speech, personality and sensory and motor functions reside. If you think of the artery as a hollow tube within another tube, the blood flows through the inner one. Now when the artery tears, the tissue on the inner wall separates allowing the blood to flow outside of the inner wall. The only way they usually tear is when they are subjected to blunt trauma. Being hit over the head by a cricket bat could do the trick, or being in a high impact car crash. It's not all that often that the intra-cranial carotid artery dissects, being a spontaneous tear with no apparent cause is quite rare.

At the most, this gave reason as to why my head was causing me so much grief. Reasons as to why those elephants had decided to take up permanent residence in my head. But they weren't exactly answers, they just paved the way for more questions. It was obviously going to be a long journey ahead.

Many of the tests that followed were to find out why this had happened. The stroke wasn't a major concern. Okay at age 31, having a stroke is a little concern, but the main concern was the dissection. According to my neurologist I was very lucky. Apparently the morbidity rate on this is quite high. It also appears that this type of dissection is more commonly seen in major head trauma. Of which I had none. I think I would have remembered having my head smashed in at some point. But no, in my case it was a spontaneous dissection. Something that doesn't normally happen to anybody. So why, why did it happen? How did it happen? What caused this? Test after test and no answers. Things like this don't just happen, there is a reason for everything, surely?

With not many answers and having the inquisitive mind that I had, I wanted to know more, needed to know more. Nothing was coming back to shed any light on the subject. From the professor down in London, to my local neurologist and all his friends. Everyone was drawing blanks. What if this were to happen again? Would I be so lucky next time? There just had to be some sort of reason, something I could do so I could somehow avoid a repeat occurrence and keep myself safe.

So the next part of my adventure, I call it an adventure, although not really sure that is what I should call it. Maybe a journey? Perhaps you'd class adventures as having a some sort of excitement. If this is an adventure, then its not really exciting, more mind boggling with a hint of scariness. But hey ho, it is what it is.

Armed with a little time and the power of Google, I decided it was time to see what I could come up with. I strongly believe that with the right attitude then anything can be accomplished. I believe that everything has a reasoning behind it. Although at first we may never know that reason, but all will become clear and work out in the end. I've always been good at figuring things out, learning from careful study how things work. If my mind was focused enough then the potential to do anything is within our grasp. The impossible can become possible and any hurdle can become overcome.

With a cup of Tetleys finest tea in hand, pyramid style I might add, I sat myself down in front of the keyboard and looked at my screen. The Google search engine staring back at me. The rainbow colours of each letter glaring at me with the cursor flashing in the search box before me. What exactly was I looking for and where would I start? I'm not sure I knew, but I was going to give it a try and see what happened. Much like I'm doing now, just going with the flow.

As my fingers began to type, entering the most obvious choice first:

spontaneous intra-cranial carotid dissection

As good as any place to start right? This search came up with a number of links. So away I begin clicking. The first link led me to a page explaining exactly what it was. I kind of already knew this. I had the explanation in layman's terms as to what it was from various people. There was a tear in the wall of the artery, and apparently for the intra-cranial artery to dissect was very uncommon. It tended to be more the extra cranial one that this happened to if any. There were also various pictures of brains and veins looking like leeches. Nice, but not what I wanted to look at, I wanted the cause, or at least some idea of a cause.

A few more searches later, after reading more information I came upon a case study report. You have to be careful what you read online when doing this type of thing, you can often shock yourself and read things that you don't want to hear. Much of the information is old hat, figures are out of date, so you have to syphon through a lot of it, using your common sense as some sort of logical filter. I knew in the back of my mind there was going to be a lot of reading involved, a lot of cups of tea, and the probability that I wouldn't find anything. After all, the greatest minds in the country were working on this for me, so surely I wouldn't be able to do any better than them! Or could I?

So this case study report I was looking at. It was a little hidden in the depths of Google's search engines results, I remember it not being on the first page, or the second, but somewhere further along on maybe the third or fourth page. As I clicked through it, once again reading all the blah de blah this and blah de blah that, I didn't think it would lead anywhere. However, just as I was about to move on I saw something regarding possible causes. There were two reasons as to why a spontaneous dissection could occur. The second I couldn't tell you what it was, as going back now my memory fails me. It often does nowadays, but like I say, a lot of things have happened in the past few years. The first reason was simply typed out in three letters:

E.D.S

My eyes focused on those letters, as if they were jumping out in front of me, dancing on the screen and shouting at me to have a look. Of course they weren't actually moving, but then I was a little fuelled up with coffee and tea, so in my mind they could have been!

What was E.D.S? What exactly did these three letters mean? How could they cause an artery to randomly dissect inside of my head? Had I stumbled across something that could lead to some sort of answer? What I didn't realise by stumbling upon these letters was that I was about to open a whole new can of worms. Questions that would lead to more questions, answers that could never be found!

2

Before we go into what I had just found, we are going to go for a little bit of a family history lesson. Yes, I want to tell you what I found out about EDS, but first I want to tell you another story. After that it will give you a greater insight as to why those three letters were to become so important in my life, in my families lives.

Right now it's time for my father to step into the story. I'm Dave, my son is Gordon, which you know now. I know I'm not really using a conventional method of writing, but you have to keep up, keep your mind sharp and stay with me.

My father is my hero. So's my mother, but it's not her turn yet! There's no two ways about that. To me he is an immortal being who defies all logic, defies all medical science and fights through anything that is put in his way. He moans a lot, he talks to himself, he comes out with the strangest of crap, much like me I guess, but above all else he is a rock. Stronger than ox. He is a walking medical mystery who has had so many problems that it is more than a miracle that he is still with us.

When my father, Howard for namesake, was around the age of 37, he had his first heart attack. He wasn't a smoker, he didn't drink a great deal, well no more than any other hard working guy. He used to work in a lace curtain factory, I don't remember a lot, but he worked long hours so that we could have a comfortable enough life. We never really wanted for a great deal, we being my younger sister and my older brother. He was also a bit of a fisherman, having his own boat and often venturing out just off the shores, laying crab pots and such like.

Well, at the time of his first heart attack, after all his investigations were carried out it turned out he had this inheritable condition called Hypertrophic Cardiomyopathy. HCM for short, much easier to remember like that. It is basically a thickening of the heart. The heart will pump blood in, but won't pump blood out at the same rate due to the thickening, or vice versa. At the time he was also told that he would be lucky if he lived for another five years. Obviously he defied this, as he's still here today, sat in my parents front room, and probably right now sat there watching some old WW2 documentaries. Since my brother moved to Germany, father had become slightly obsessed with the place and its history. A healthy obsession mind!

After many complications and more heart attacks later, angina attacks, kidney stones, there's a whole long list of ailments in there. Maybe I shall list them at the back of the book, I'm sure it would take a whole page in itself, we come to a little time after I had my dissection. My dissection was in the August, and this occurrence I believe was either in the November of 2011 or the February of 2012. It doesn't really matter. It happened and that's all there is to it. The point is, what happened was about to tie in with my investigations.

Another normal day. The sun had been shining, casting a little warmth onto what was slightly chilly weather. What was about to happen this day was going to test us all, push us to places that tore out our hearts, tested us mentally and physically, and forge a bond between us that no words can describe. Another great darkness was about to creep upon all of us, to try and break us, but stand fast we would do.

As I recall, my father was sat at the computer desk and talking to someone on the phone, who this someone was I do not know. All I remember was that he was sat there in that chair. He put the phone down, then went to stand up, but as he stood up, he cried out in pain. A pain of which I cannot describe, as this time it wasn't me feeling it. I can only imagine it must have been that invisible knife being driven deep inside, cutting through the flesh and twisting. Back down on the chair he slumped, trying to hide the pain he was in, but the look in his eyes said it all, the beads of sweat appearing on his forehead said it all. This wasn't his usual chest pain, this was the onset of something more sudden, something that caused him to reel back, a pain to the left side of the stomach which was unlike anything he had had before. And yes he had pain before, he had known pain like it was his friend, I'd seen his pain before and it scared me, but this was different.

Managing to get to his feet after the sharpness subsided a little he made it to the bedroom to lie down. The sweat was pouring off him. His face had turned grey, all trace of normal colour washed out. He lay there writhing in agony, sickness taking over. It was time to call for an ambulance yet again.

My mother, Gertrude, had called the ambulance. The conversation was quick, with urgency in her voice. The ambulance needed to get here fast, which it didn't. This is Lincolnshire and nothing happens fast in Lincolnshire. For the next 45 minutes, maybe slightly more, my father lay in that bedroom rolling around in agony, being sick, sweating and groaning in pain. It didn't subside, it didn't go away, whatever this was it was relentless in its torment. It was like a crazed starved animal feeding on its latest meal, ripping it to shreds like a maniac.

The ambulance eventually turned up. It seemed like an age but at last it was here and help had arrived. I don't know what happened in that bedroom, for there wasn't enough room to be anywhere near, but they put him in the ambulance that had pulled right up the drive and to the side of the house so as not to move him far.

Onwards to hospital it went, with us in tow, a procession of cars following the ambulance that contained my father. It's speed wasn't great, it couldn't have been for every single bump, my father would have felt it like that knife stabbing him over and over again. The roads around here are not the best, potholes everywhere, to go at any speed would be a disaster.

Upon arrival at the hospital he was taken straight into Accident and Emergency, and given pain relief after being initially checked over. It took a while but then he was transferred to another part of the hospital. It was another ward not unlike the one I had been in, only this time I believe it was something to do with surgical assessment. We hadn't been told much at this point, apart from the fact he was waiting for a CT scan, which was going to be a while. The pain had subsided a little due to the pain killers, and sleep had embraced him. I only hoped that he was a little more comfortable in his sleep.

Time went by slowly, and things seemed to be calming down a little. We spoke to the nurses and they said that they were waiting for a doctor to come round and were waiting to get him sent down for the CT. They advised us to go and get a coffee and a sandwich while we waited, which we did. They had our phone numbers, and would call if anything came to light, and he was asleep so reluctantly off we went.

Of course we couldn't really eat, the effects of seeing the ones you love and care about being in so much pain somehow makes you lose your appetite. The feeling of being powerless to do anything about it racks up an anger inside of you. It fuels the darkness inside that builds up, but a coffee would be had, a strong one at that. But then it wasn't that strong being from one of those vending machines in the lobby. In fact it even tasted a bit like the cardboard cup that it was sat in. I will give the coffee 10 out of 10 for being hot though, singed lips were often the case with these vending machine coffees. I think someone needs to look into inventing something to rectify this.

Meanwhile, coffees finished, and a little time spent in the lobby watching the hustle and bustle of people walking backwards and forwards, we headed off back upstairs. Myself, my mother and my sister. All unaware off what was about to be said to us. Not prepared in any way, shape or form. The lift ride up was full of people but completely silent. Often this was the case; no-one ever really talks inside these confined spaces. Metallic boxes clunking as they rise floor after floor. Not one person held inside wanted to be here, who wants to be in a hospital, there are no good points about being in hospital. The only time you come to a hospital is when someone is unwell.

As we reached our floor we disembarked from our silent ride. First my mother, then my sister, then myself, once again a left turn out of the lift then another left turn down the long wide corridor. My mothers footsteps echoing down the corridor with every step, mine giving a little rubbery screech against the shiny floor, which I'd never to do on purpose to make light of the situation obviously!

Coming up to my father's room at the end of the corridor on the right, we were stopped just outside of the door by an oldish fair haired nurse.

"We have been trying to reach you" she said in a soft voice. I found they often did this when they had something not so nice to say.

"My phone has been switched on but it hasn't rung" my mother replied.

As she was speaking, I could see into my father's room. There was a doctor and a surgeon at the end of the bed, talking to him.

"Well never mind you're here now."

As the nurse said this she began to reach up and place her hand on my mothers shoulder.

"Howard has been for his CT scan, the doctor is with him now, I'm afraid it's not good news."

"What do you mean?" came my mothers reply, as all three sets of our eyes locked onto the nurse and what she was about to tell us.

"We need to transfer Howard to a more specialised hospital straight away, he's had the CT scan and it has shown a dissection on the superior mesenteric artery."

Her voice was even softer now, sympathetic even. But there it was, that dissection word again. Coincidence, perhaps not I thought.

"So what are you saying?" I blurted out.

Her reply was straight to the point.

"It's time to hope for the best."

"What, he's going to die?"

"If we don't get him to Lincoln and operated on it is highly likely."

"I have a son who lives in Germany, what should we do?" came my mother, with a hint of worry in her voice.

"You should call him and if he can get here he might want to come." With that reply the seriousness of the situation impacted our minds. I could see the pain in my mother's eyes, in my sister's eyes. I could feel my own eyes beginning to fill with the salty water that tears bring, but I wasn't going to let that be seen here, not yet, there's a time and a place.

With that the nurse took us into the room where my father was. The surgeon and the doctor walked out past us and we walked in. They didn't say a word, they didn't even acknowledge our presence, instead they walked past us with their heads pointed down to the ground.

As we closed into my father's bed, I could see his eyes were filled with tears. He looked over at us with what looked like great sorrow. There were no words, nothing could describe this moment. The harsh reality of what perhaps we had tried to prepare ourselves for all our lives. I can't say how anyone else felt, all I knew were my own feelings, but what I felt was indescribable. With no amount of preparation can you ready yourself for something like this. We always knew that eventually this day would come, but not today, not now. My heart felt like it was being ripped apart, a pain so terrifying, a torture so sadistic. Right now I would rather be one of those guys in the Saw films, stuck in one of those bizarre traps, anything to be away from here and not have to feel the hurt that was pulling me apart at the seams. But it was real, and it was happening.

What followed was a lot of hugging, a few tears, and even a few "I love yous" which didn't really need to be said. We all knew the score, this was looking like the end.

"Ring your brother" came the quiet broken voice, from the once immortal being.

3

My sister, Franny … that's right Franny, you heard right. So a quick recap, I'm Dave, my son's Gordon, my dad is Howard, my mum is Gertrude and my sister is Franny. It's good you're keeping up my friends and yes reader I now am beginning to class you as my friend. I would be wrong not to, as you are entering the thoughts that I have kept locked away at the back of mind. You are learning about me and my experiences like no other. I hope you feel special, as I don't talk about these things often!

Franny and I headed back downstairs, leaving my mother with my father to wait for the ambulance for the transferral. When we got downstairs I had to compose myself. What we were about to do was make the long distance phone call to Germany. Not a phone call anybody would want to make. But it had to be done. So a cigarette was lit to calm the nerves, but then there weren't any really, it was as if I was in a trance, I didn't really feel anything, as if it wasn't happening. It was all some kind of bizarre nightmare. Surely any minute now I would wake up back in my own bed and it would be over. If only that were the case.

I reached into my jacket pocket, my leather jacket pocket I might add, that's how I was rolling today, in my hard ass leathers. I pulled out that swanky smartphone I mentioned a while back, brought up the menu for contacts, and there he was, brother Charlie. The Englishman that had gone German. Lifting the phone to my ear I made the call, breathing in deeply as it rang to keep my cool calm composure.

"Hello" came the voice from a million miles away, well not that far, Germany remember.

"Hi it's Dave." Of course he knew who it was, my voice hadn't changed that much, but in these circumstances I may have sounded a little different.

"How you doing? What's wrong?" Charlie could obviously hear a distinct change in my voice. Perhaps that undertone of desperation.

"Its ..." trying to keep myself in check I cleared my throat.

"Its … Dad, he's in hospital, he's ..." with that I let out a sort of wounded yelp like a puppy having it's toes stood on.

"What, what's wrong?"

There was now an urgency in Charlie's voice.

Calmness had left the building. A wave of emotion hit me like a ton of bricks. My eyes welled up and tears began to roll down my cheeks.

"They say he's had a dissection, a tear in one of his arteries near his stomach" I blurted it out quickly like I was sneezing it out.

"What, like you had?"

"Yes, the same but in a different place."

"Is he okay?"

To this there was only one answer.

"No ..." halting for a moment, I took a deep breath, "They say he might not make it, they say they need to transfer him to another hospital to have an operation otherwise he might not make it, they told us to hope for the best."

And that was it, the tears were coming full force. I felt Franny throw her arms around me. We stood there in silence, just holding on to each other, the phone still at my ear but no words coming through. I can only assume my words were sinking in. Doing this in a phone call was not the way it should have been, but being so far away it was the only way it could be done. Then came the reply.

"I'm coming over, how long do we have? Will I make it in time?"

"I'm not sure, we are waiting for the ambulance, just be careful and drive safely."

"I'll get there, it's nine here now, I'll get there by morning, I'll find a ferry to come across on and I'll get there, I'll meet you there. I'll ring when I get to England, if anything changes then let me know."

And after that the phone went down. I could only hope that he was careful. The last thing we wanted was for Charlie to come flying here like a madman and end up in a accident along the way somewhere.

This is where that sub story ends. Because you know, my father is still sat there in his chair, making those silly comments that only he could make, watching his morbid documentaries on WW2, and all things Hitler. Spying on the people of Germany on the town based street cams. Remember, our Howard is an immortal being who defies all medical knowledge and fights with every ounce of his being to stay alive. He doesn't give up, he never will. A true warrior who goes on and on forever.

My brother made it across the waters on his monstrous trek; I'm sure that's another story in itself, an adventure, these little adventures that life puts in our paths for us to battle through. When my father got to the other hospital, yes, they said he needed an operation or he would die, but then they said they couldn't do it as it was too risky and he would probably not wake up. Instead, they left him to fight it himself, to hope for the best and pray that he would be able to get through this. Of course in this dark time, we did not lose hope, and he did not stop fighting. The night was one of the longest I have ever known. Going from needing an emergency surgical intervention, to being left to his own devices. The risks were too great for anyone to willingly intervene. The fight for life was left to him and only him, and by some miracle he prevailed. Miraculously, his body would come to heal itself.

So take a little time to reflect on that one, it wasn't an easy piece for me to write. I would have rather put that one away in a little box in my mind and kept it locked away forever. However, as it turns out, I feel this story is now more about facing our inner demons. I'm beginning to realise more and more you can't just hide everything inside. You have to face the darkness, face your fears before they devour you.

If you're sticking with this, then you should probably have noticed that the dissection thing keeps cropping up. Once in myself and now in my father. There's a pattern forming here, two generations suffering from the same problem, now as you will see, this is where the relevance of those three letters begins to take shape … E.D.S.

4

Back to Google and back to being sat in front of my computer screen. The endless cups of tea and coffee flowing through my system making me need to urinate over and over again. Like I said, I knew this wasn't going to be easy, but it seemed like I might now being getting somewhere, so another search was in order.

Placing my hands once again over the keyboard, I started to type into the box of searchfulness, "EDS symptoms". What that search result brought back was a whole list of links, one after the other. The common thing with all these links was that those letters now had a meaning. There on the page before me, endless websites with:

Ehlers-Danlos Syndrome

Out of all the links I really didn't know which one to choose. I guess it didn't matter, so it was gonna be a case of pot luck and lets see what it brings back. I scrolled down the page a little, reading the subtext I found one of interest and clicked on it. Don't ask me why, I just felt a little more drawn to it than to any of the others. It just sort of happened, as things have a tendency to do.

What came up next appeared to be a a reasonably simple website, pretty straightforward and easy to read. I was on a page that had a sub heading of "*Vascular type EDS*". Reading the first line, it suddenly dawned on me that luck, if you can call it that, may have pointed me in the right direction. What was written there made me pause for a minute.

The Vascular type of EDS is characterized by possible arterial or organ rupture as a result of spontaneous rupture of vessels or organs due to the result of even minor trauma. The Vascular type of EDS is the most serious form of Ehlers-Danlos Syndrome.

Thinking for a minute it made a little sense. Arterial rupture, spontaneous. A dissection was similar to a rupture in that it was a tear in the inner arterial wall as opposed to the outer arterial wall, and being spontaneous it just happens? With no reason, like in my head, like in my father?

Not wanting to get too far ahead of myself and come to any assumptions I carried on reading. There were a few bits and pieces of information that I wasn't really interested in right now, so I skimmed a little past it all, not really paying a lot of attention until I came to another sub heading:

Clinical diagnosis

Okay, so this is perhaps what I was looking for. Symptoms. I figured there was no point in looking and learning about something unless I knew that there definitely could be a relevance to me. There were two sections to this. There was a major diagnostic criteria and a minor diagnostic criteria. According to the write up, if you you ticked two of the major criteria then it was strongly recommended to get your ass tested. With the minor criteria, ticking one or more of the boxes would lead to supporting that theory.

My eyes flowed down the page to look at the major diagnostic criteria. There were four bullet points, out of the four, there were two staring me in the face.

Arterial rupture. I had established that the dissection was the similar to a rupture, due to weakness in the arterial wall. So yes, that's one major box ticked.

Family history of the vascular type of EDS. This one was a little more complicated, I'd never heard of this before. No-one had, but logic depicts, my father and I had both had dissections. My grandmother and great grandmother on my father's side died of an aneurysm at at an early age. This was all do with veins and arteries, the vascular system. Perhaps this was all linked? So in a fashion another box ticked.

Eager to know more, excited if you like, I went ever further down to take a look at the minor diagnostic criteria. This list contained a lot more bullet points.

Easy bruising (spontaneous or with minimal trauma.) This was a definite tick. All my life I had bruised easily. My legs and arms would always have some sort of bruise on them. I couldn't always explain where they came from as half the time I never even remembered knocking myself. Of course all these years I had never thought anything of it. It didn't really cause me any problems and it seemed normal to me. There was the odd time that someone mentioned it, but I never really paid attention, why would I? My father was the same, so was my sister, it was the way it was. Until now that is!

Characteristic facial appearance (thin lips and philtrum, small chin, thin nose, large eyes.) Another one for the tick box perhaps. Not a definite but a perhaps. My lips are a little on the thin side I suppose, and if you remember me saying, if had shaved my goatee off, then my chin would disappear, so I guess you could say I had a small chin, and as for the large eyes, people had also remarked that I have big brown eyes in the past. A little sceptical on this one, but enough to pass for another tick.

Hypermobility of small joints. I had never thought of myself as being flexible. In fact I wasn't. But upon looking at my hands, the tips of my fingers all bend back. It turns out that most peoples don't. I have one that doesn't bend back, it's as about as straight as you can get, but the rest all bend back slightly further. Again this is something that I classed as normal and just assumed everything else was the same. Apparently not, perhaps my body was a little different.

My gut feeling told me that there was obviously something in this. I still didn't really know what this Vascular Ehlers-Danlos thing was, but was beginning to think that it could maybe unlock a few mysteries. I didn't want to delve into it too far, but knew if I was to pursue this then I would need to be armed with just a little bit more information.

Back to the Google search box we went for one final time this evening. I say evening, the evening had now slipped away, and the darkness of the night was giving way to the rising of the sun. The birds had began their morning song. Time had passed away quickly without me realising. I had been so caught up in searching for answers that time had lost its meaning. I was just slurping on my tea, obviously you have to have a little slurp, you know, place your top lip so it just sits in the tea, then give it a gentle suck in. I'm sure this releases the flavours, wouldn't you agree?

The cursor in my box was winking at me, eagerly waiting for me to work my fingers once again. It was like playing a game of fetch with a loyal companion of the four legged type. I think we had made a connection, pretty much like you and I. My fingers hovered over once again, and gave life to my winking friend. **Vascular Ehler-Danlos Syndrome**. And fetch!

Being the loyal companion he was, immediately brought back to me was another list of links full of the words Ehlers-Danlos Syndrome. The second link down was my link of choice. It was a support page based here in the UK. "Great" I thought to myself, this could be an interesting lesson.

I was now beginning to learn that Ehlers-Danlos Syndrome was a group of inheritable disorders, which affects the connective tissues in our bodies. More importantly it affected the production of the collagen. In layman's terms, collagen is a kind of a glue. It bonds us together, much like the foundations of a house. If the foundations of a house are faulty, it can lead to all sorts of problems, cracks appear, the house can fall down. Well this is the same with collagen, if it's faulty, cracks appear within us. Not just in once place, but anywhere. Seeing as collagen is found almost anywhere in our bodies, the possibilities are endless.

It appeared that there were many types of Ehlers-Danlos Syndrome. Seven sub types had been named in total. All different in their being, yet all having similar connections. I briefly looked through a few of the different types and as I did it became clear that the vascular type was definitely the way to go if any. It was going to be a long shot, as it was rarer than most types, 1 in 250,000 were the figures. Perhaps the one thing that stuck in mind the most was that the vascular type was the most life threatening. But of course if this was it, I already knew, as it had tried to get me once already, and many times my father had danced with the devil. There was also no known cure, no known treatment. It was random in its nature.

That was it, I was growing weary and beginning to read things that I didn't really want to know about yet. One step at a time.

5

Once more into the fray we go. With the information I had acquired I had to decide the route on which to take it forward. Did I wait and see my neurologist? Sure he was a nice man, but old and set in his ways. Maybe he was approachable in that way but with age comes stubbornness. This man, it came to light, had treated my granddad years ago. He had also seen my father, so had knowledge of my family. But would he think maybe that I was belittling him if I took this information to him? I didn't want it to come across that way, I wanted to help in the investigations not make anyone feel like I was sticking my nose in. I had to play this one very carefully, I wanted to be taken seriously, have a proper discussion about my findings. To be able to talk about it rather than be shot down before I had even started. If after discussing it, I was laughed at and told not to be silly, then that would be okay. It's rare, I knew this about it and it was a long shot!

With those thoughts in mind, I started to think about the young doctor. I had now seen her on quite a few occasions, and remembering that initial gut feeling I believed this would be the way to go. I remembered how every time I saw her, she sat there and looked me straight in the eye, listening and taking in every word that came out of my mouth. Yes, she would be the one.

Picking up the phone once again I made the call, and got the appointment. Armed with my piece of paper and a tick list, I went down to the surgery.

Sitting outside her room again now, the wait this time was long. The place was busy, everyone was running behind. I was feeling quite nervous about what exactly I was going to say and how exactly I was going to say it. I didn't want to risk putting anyone's back up. Perhaps I shouldn't have felt like this, perhaps I should have more faith, but it's the way it was. I didn't exactly feel confident in my ability, after all the people I'd been to see. Surely it should have been one of them to come up with some answers, not from me, sat searching the internet with Google as my weapon. I began again counting the ticking seconds.

"1 1000, 1 2000 .."

Hmm I'd been here many times before now, but then came that voice through the air,

"David Malarky to see Dr Haramesh."

And with that I politely knocked on the door, you must never just barge in remember, manners are manners!

"Good morning David."

Her eyes locked onto me and her smile was wide, could it be possible that she was pleased to see me?

"Good morning."

My reply was a little timid with a hint of nervousness in there. As I took to my seat next to her, I reached into my pocket to pull out the crumpled piece of paper with my check list on it.

"I hope you don't mind me coming in here like this, but I've been doing a little research and I seem to have stumbled across something which may or may not have some relevance to everything that's been going on." With that I began to unravel the paper a little.

"Okay, that's good" was the unexpected reply I got, her eyes looking deep into mine and down at the paper with great interest.

"I came across something called Ehlers-Danlos Syndrome, Vascular Ethler-Danlos Syndrome to be more accurate. After reading about it, it turns out it can cause arterial ruptures, and its an inheritable condition."

As I broke out into all the different criteria Dr Haramesh listened tentatively. I seemed to be getting my point across and she was nodding in agreement to what I had to say. A little relief flowed through me and I felt a little more at ease and confident in what I was doing. I always knew my gut instinct was right, and I should not have worried that it would be taken the wrong way.

After a long discussion, it was decided that yes, this could actually be a possibility. There was a valid case as to why this should be looked at. It was too early to tell if this could possibly be the cause of a history of one families' problems. But what you couldn't ignore was that the facts were there, staring you in the face. Small things which had been overlooked over the years, the bigger picture never really being noticed. Now the pieces of the jigsaw were coming together. The road however would still be long, challenges still lie ahead. For myself, I didn't realise it then, but my greatest challenge was just beginning. Without even realising it, the darkness that would grow inside of me was being fuelled.

"Our next step then is to get into contact with a genetics team. I will write off to them for you regarding what we have discussed today, it might take a while but we shall see what happens."

Her voice was one of sympathy, and pleasurable warmth.

"Thank you for your help."

I arose from my seat and made the journey home.

6

Time began to go by. On this path I was now following there were no short cuts, there was no way to speed things up. The pain in my head eventually subsided, I would still occasionally get the migraines but they began to drift off. After a while I went back to work and life pretty much flowed quite nicely. For now I locked away the thoughts of this Vascular Ehlers-Danlos Syndrome. There was no point really thinking about any of the consequences it could unravel. There was no point learning about it, it wasn't yet a reality, and maybe it wouldn't become a reality. However even though it was locked away, times would still come when it would niggle away at me.

Of course there were still problems. Nothing at my

end, but my father again had another dissection. It was more or less the same as last time. Not only once did we go through the experience, but no, it came again. We were told that he wouldn't make it, but obviously being the immortal being that he is, he did. For some reason the medical community, even after all these years, doesn't seem to realise that our family doesn't just roll over and die. It's not in our blood, we are born fighters against all odds, we never give in in times of trouble. Sure we may stumble, and yes we stumble hard, but we always hang on to that small glimmer of hope, and in the end we pull through.

While we are waiting around for that appointment to come, yes I had to wait, quite a while, so I'm going make you wait too, Give a little, take a little, life is a two way street. This story is on pause for a while. Come over here, lets have a little chat. I'd like to talk about Gertrude. You do know who Gertrude is? Okay lets have a quick recap, you might get this you might not, but if you have ever watched "Blind Date" with Cilla Black back in the 90's …

"Here's our Graham with a quick recap!"

Don't forget to say it in that Liverpudlian accent of hers!

So … we have myself, Dave or David if you really prefer, we have my son Gordon, we have my father Howard, my mother Gertrude, my sister Franny and my brother the German defector Charlie. We are the Malarky family and "Family Fortunes" this is not … "Catchphrase" however, now there's a programme! I don't mean to insult anyone's intelligence here, but I do feel its good to have a refresh every now and then. It's a complicated yarn, emotional, twisty, exciting, dark and hopeful. You are also delving inside the deepest part of my mind, so it may get a little confusing at times! A little light hearted distraction I would say is definitely needed with such a serious subject matter.

Gertrude, ah yes, my mother. What can I say about her? Well again where to start? She is my mother, so obviously I am a little biased, however I could not wish for a better mother than her. She is a ray of sunshine. She is a legend. You see, through all the ailments that my father Howard has seen, she has been there by his side. She has been beside him in every ounce of pain. I believe that when you love someone, you go through everything they go through. Maybe not physically, but mentally and emotionally you feel it.

Through all these many times, and there have been many, too many to talk about here; for that we would have to write an epic saga, she has stuck by him. Not only that, she has been there for us, myself, Franny and Charlie. We have all had our episodes of causing great chaos in our parent's lives, but they remain there, not judging, but supporting. By our sides in whatever we do. Gertrude's head is strong, transfixed on positivity. Full of love, caring, considerate and kind. Anyone who has ever met my mother has always commented on how nice she is, and they're right, she is. She has time and space in her heart for anyone! Personally I like to think that I have got a little of her in me. Having a tiny shred of what she has in me makes me a better person. Keeps me headstrong, keeps me positive, and gives me the love that I have in my heart.

And while we are at it, should we not introduce Franny? I think we should. My dear sister, what can I say about her. I can say she doesn't like her name too much. But it is such a good name, Franny! That name just makes you smile! In reality though, my sister, another great warrior of the Malarky tribe. Franny has great strength. From being knocked down she has risen to great heights. In the literal sense, as we speak she is probably planning her next mountain climb. Over the last few years she has been doing a lot of charity work for a road safety charity. This has taken her up the Mount of Snowdon against all odds, and she has pushed forward and her courage has shone through. A true inspiration to us all, spreading joy to many people's lives. One thing though, she does have a dislike of werewolves, and I really don't know why that is!

Then we come to the defector Charlie. What on earth was he thinking leaving this land of green and pleasant pastures. I'm not so sure myself, but he's gone out there on his own, from having nothing, to building a life in a foreign land. That my friends takes some balls of steel. To leave everything you know, to go out there with nothing and to build up from scratch in a place you know not of. It takes great courage. It takes strength. But he's gone and done it, a good job, a nice house and even a little baby girl on the way. Nothing but total respect, and he's always there when needed. He drove all those miles at the drop of hat, and was here when needed most even when he was so far away.

Yes, so now you know my immediate family a little. Hopefully things are beginning to become a little clearer now as to what this story is really about. My mind does drift, but like I said I'm not your conventional story teller. I'm no Stephen King, I'm no Dean Koontz. I'm just plain old Dave!

7

So back we come to the story at hand, to continue on with the journey. A few more months had passed by. Nothing really interesting had happened. Dr Haramesh had been true to her word and had set the wheels in motion. In the May of 2013, just after my 33rd birthday, I received a phone call from the Ehlers-Danlos clinic. I had been told previously that this phone call was coming, through copies of letters backwards and forwards from my GP. The idea behind it was to have a phone interview. Now the EDS clinic is a very busy place. It deals with all things genetic, and only has a small team, so their time is precious. The idea of the phone call, from what I believed, was to see if it what I had found did really hold any weight behind it.

During the phone call, we went through everything that had happened to me during my time of the elephants. We took a stroll down memory lane and went back to my childhood. If I'm honest I don't remember my childhood that well, whether this was something caused by the stroke or the dissection I do not know. Maybe my memory is just shit? But we regressed a little and I answered questions on what I could remember. Now I've always thought that there was something slightly odd about me, well I know there is mentally, but my gut feeling, and remember my gut feeling is usually right, told me that my body had always been a little different. I just didn't realise how different it really was.

Through our stroll down memory lane, we talked about bruising, which as I had said before, I always seemed to have a lot of bruises, and throughout life this had never changed. The slightest knock and I would have bruises that lasted for weeks, not always being able to explain where they came from. Up until now I had thought this was normal, but it seems not. We talked about how my veins would burst, especially on my feet. If I walked around in bare feet or in socks, then at some point I would feel a pinch on the bottom of my foot, then it would itch, the vein would be bulging out on my sole, causing me to be unable to walk with my foot flat. Also, about how the veins would burst in my legs, my wrists. Again no reason for it, I didn't even have to knock them, they would just spontaneously burst, leaving me sore and bruised. All these little things were quite normal to me.

We then went on to talk about my activities, how I fared with exercise. When I was around the age of 15-16 I used to go to kick boxing. I loved it with a passion. It gave me focus, discipline. I used to train one night a week, but that was enough. Obviously a sport like this is not easy on anyone's body, but now the pieces were being put together I began to realise why I found it even harder. A simple, straightforward roundhouse kick would make my hip feel like it was popping, and the warm up sit-ups would make me feel like my stomach muscles were being torn apart. By the time the night was over, I would be in pain, it would be hard to walk, my muscles would ache, my joints would hurt and it took a few days to recover. I thought this was normal. I know the training was hard, but I thought I was feeling the same as everyone else. It turns out it wasn't.

A few years ago, I went with a few friends to a giant paint ball match. "North vs. South" it was called. It was a big full day's worth of a game, around 1200 players in total. A long day, a lot of walking, crouching and a little bit of running. I wasn't the fittest of people, but I also wouldn't have classed myself as unfit. I was active daily, doing physical work. So by the end of the day I could hardly walk, and my thigh muscles were causing me great pain. Every step I took felt like they were being shredded apart. I had to walk up steps sideways, as my muscles couldn't take going up just one step properly. Sure, everyone else ached, and I wasn't any less fit than they were. I hadn't walked twice as far as they had, but I felt like I had ran four marathons in one day. After that it took a whole week to be able to walk properly again, when everyone else was back to normal in just a couple of days. I'd never really known any different, so again, I thought this was all normal.

After going through my history, we looked into that of my father's, and all the problems that he had encountered. Obviously I couldn't list them all, there were too many for that. His bruisings were the same, his veins were the same, his dissections, we talked about how no-one had looked any further beyond the Hypertrophic Cardiomyopathy. We talked about his mother, and how if you touched her she would bruise, how her veins would burst, how she died of an aneurysm at an early age. With this phone call, a picture was being painted, pieces were being placed together and mysteries were being unravelled.

When the phone call was over, it was quite clear that all the little things that I had always thought were normal, well they weren't. Something wasn't quite right with my body, with my fathers body, and as we would soon come to find out, my sisters body too. Vascular Ehlers-Danlos Syndrome seemed to hold the key. Now I had been invited over to see the geneticists, but first we would once again have to play the waiting game. But that appointment would be coming.

8

Days and weeks again passed by. From time to time I would think about this Vascular Ehlers-Danlos Syndrome. Still no appointment had come through and I had heard nothing more. My mind was growing curious. I started to want to know what this thing was that I had found. All roads were now pointing in this direction. My inquisitive mind was getting the better of me, and although I may have been jumping the gun a little, I had to know more.

Over the course of the next few days I spent many an hour doing research, searching here and there for every little bit of information I could find. I read about it, I watched videos on YouTube about it, I looked in forums. Hunting high and low, I was gathering information like a little squirrel scurrying for nuts. I was becoming obsessed in feeding my knowledge. There was a small problem with this though. There really wasn't a lot of information out there. Most of the pages I found, most of the information I found, was going over the same old thing time and time again repeating itself like a stuck record. Some of the information was old, some of it even conflicted. The truth is that there wasn't enough known about Vascular Ehlers-Danlos to have complete figures and facts. Although it had been around for many many years, the documentation on it was very minimal due to its rareness, and due to the fact that a lot of people over the years had gone undiagnosed. The most common form of Ehlers-Danlos Syndrome seemed to be type 3. This type was classed as hypermobility. Although still classed as rare, there seemed to be a large community, but I wasn't interested in it one bit. Whilst yes, it was part of the syndrome, Vascular Ehlers-Danlos was a breed unto itself.

To tell you exactly what Vascular Ehlers-Danlos Syndrome is doesn't take a lot. Whilst it causes many problems throughout the entire body (remember it's a defect of the collagen that is found everywhere in our body) and is very complex and random in its nature, it's summing up is pretty simple. So with the help of the material that I did find I shall explain:

Vascular Ehlers-Danlos Syndrome is recognized to be the most severe form of EDS. It is a life threatening connective tissue disorder that affects all tissues and internal organs making them extremely fragile. It is

also very uncommon and it is estimated to account for less than 5% of the EDS population.

Vascular Ehlers-Danlos patients are at risk of sudden arterial or organ rupture. This can occur at any age. Arterial rupture accounts for the majority of death in vascular EDS and any artery can be affected, although 50% occur in the chest and abdomen, 25% in the head and neck and the rest in the extremities.

A quarter of individuals experience a significant medical complication by age 20 years and more than 80% by the age of 40 years.

During the latter stages of pregnancy severe complications such as rupture of the uterus (womb) may occur, but this is fortunately relatively uncommon. Premature births due to cervical insufficiency (weakness) and foetal membrane fragility are seen in Vascular EDS, as well as in the other EDS types.

Partial collapse of the lungs (pneumothorax) is more frequent in individuals with Vascular EDS and affects about 15%. It may present with sudden shortness of breath or chest pain.

So really in a nutshell that was Vascular Ehlers-Danlos Syndrome. This was perhaps the monster lurking within that we were are facing. From the accounts that I read it was random in its very nature. The complications varied from person to person. It follows no rules, it has the ability to attack you at any point and almost anywhere, and there was little that you could do about it. There was no cure, and no real treatment, just monitoring. To perform surgery on a patient with

Vascular Ehlers-Danlos Syndrome seems to come with great risk. It had been done, but surgical intervention was not recommended unless the situation was life threatening.

Finding this out scared me, it brought fear to the forefront of my mind. Fear of the unknown. But yet there was still hope. Although everything was leading down this path, there was still that chance that it wouldn't come to pass. This was perhaps the utmost worse case scenario, I mean after all, this was just something that I stumbled on. My father had been treated over the years for many things and no-one had ever mentioned anything of the sort. He had been all over the country seeing different specialists. I had been and seen quite a few specialists myself. Surely if this was the case, then someone, one of those doctors or professors would have known about the condition, surely they would have found out by now. After nearly 25-30 years of caring for my father, someone must have surely come across it?

This was the path I had chosen to take though, I had wanted answers and I was going to get them soon enough, one way or another. I just hoped, prayed that this wasn't my answer, not just for my sake, but for everyone else's. Perhaps anything but this .. but the ball had been set and everything was in motion. It was a few weeks later that I finally came home from work and there was the letter. A brown envelope, inside containing a date and time for my appointment. Answers would shortly be coming my way.

CHAPTER 3
FAULTY FOUNDATIONS

It was now July 2013. A whole two years after my dissection and my stroke. The last couple of years had come and gone so fast. One big whirlwind of mess, sweeping us all up and pushing us along.

So much had happened in those two years, it's sometimes hard to remember the order of events. Mixed up memories and feelings. But here we were. It had been a couple of months from getting the letter to going for the appointment. Those months had been hard. I tried to put Vascular Ehlers-Danlos into a box in the back of my mind. In reality though it was always there, sub consciously lurking in the back of my mind. What if this was it. I didn't want this. Why would anyone want to feel like a ticking time bomb waiting to go off.

There were nights I would lay there, I would look back and remember that pain I had once suffered, I would look back and remember the time we were told my father was going to die, not once, but twice. Memories haunting me of the phone call I'd had to make. Something that I'm sure no-one would ever want to go through. But these incidents had come and gone, there was no point dwelling; just picking yourself up, dusting yourself off and moving forward. Life hits hard at times, but it's not about how hard you can get hit, it's about how you pull yourself back up and keep on pushing forward. It's about learning to dance in the rain.

Rising early that morning, a little after five, I had an appointment at 9:30am with the geneticists. The drive ahead of us would take two and a half hours, and we had to allow for traffic and for being able to get parked. Apparently the parking at the hospital was pretty terrible. I decided it would be best to take my father with me.

When we had been doing the family tree, I hadn't exactly been good at remembering birth dates or any of the family history to be honest. I suppose I was quite vague at best! So with this in mind, I considered it a good idea to take him with me. This would also mean they would get to see two generations of our family in one go.

Before setting off a cup of coffee was in order, my eyes were heavy, the sun hadn't yet cast it's light on our land. The birds were once again singing their morning song. There seemed to be an eerie stillness in the air, no wind. At that time of the morning the village was still sleeping, no cars going up and down the road; the bypass had put paid to that. It was peaceful, tranquil, as if the world was respecting the importance of what lay ahead.

Walking out of the house at 6:00am, the sun had begun to rise. The sky was clear, with no clouds. You could see all the morning planes criss crossing across the sky, leaving their trails painting pictures on the empty blue canvas up above. Considering how important today was, I was feeling pretty refreshed. There were no nerves, there was no fear. In fact I even felt a little content with myself. Perhaps that night I'd had an epic saga of a dream. I couldn't remember it if I did, but you know the feeling you get when you have a great dream, you wake up with a smile on your face and a feeling of contentment. That's pretty much how I felt. Maybe you think it would be a strange way to feel on a day like today, but you know I'm strange anyway!

Off we set then, onwards and over to yonder Yorkshireland. I'd not visited Sheffield in quite a few years, which I thought was quite sad really. My mother's side of the family was mostly based in Sheffield. Yes Grandad on my mothers side was Irish, but they had lived in Sheffield for years. It was my mothers place of birth, and I still had a couple of uncles living there, and a few cousins. When my grandparents were alive, there were many trips over on a regular basis. I used to spend weeks at a time staying at my grandparents, during the summer holidays as a child. It seemed a shame that it was these circumstances taking me back there. But then when you grow up time seems to slide through your fingers and you lose track, weeks turn to months, months turn to years. You tend to get caught up in the ebb of life and forget to make time for visiting your nearest and dearest. I'm sure its not just me though, I'm quite certain we are all guilty of that sometimes!

My father and I didn't say a lot on the journey there, we didn't need to really. As we were making good time we stopped halfway. Can you guess what we stopped for? I'll tell you anyway, this was a road trip, an early morning road trip. No early morning road trip can be successfully completed without a visit to McDonalds, after all, "a visit to McDonalds makes your day!" Yes, that succulent taste of a double sausage and egg mcmuffin. How can you not love those tasty little treats! The eggified smell is a little gnarly, but once you get your lips around and take a bite, wowsers what a tasty treat for breakfast! A scrumptious filling treat! And of course life is all about little treats!

With our stomachs full it was onwards with the journey. Destiny awaited us at our destination. It was pretty uneventful driving there, apart from the odd lunatic motorist who's always in a rush to get somewhere and decides to weave in and out of lanes cutting you up on the dual carriageway. We got there in one piece though, and found the place pretty easily. Parking as expected was a little on the awkward side. In front of the tall building that stood before us was a multi-storey car park that seemed to be the only apparent parking area. The time was now 8:30am and the small lane leading into it was lined with cars. As we entered we went up three storeys, tyres squealing slightly on the asphalt as we went around the tight ramps. The echoing sounds of car doors closing, as the herds of people departed and headed into the hospital. Another half an hour and I fear we wouldn't have got parked so easily!

Leaving the car we had a bit of a walk ahead of us. From the multi-storey, the entrance to the EDS clinic was all the way over the other side of the hospital. It was in a completely separate building, located inside the children's hospital. For my father the walk was hard, most of it was uphill, which was slow going with his cane. Without measuring it, it was maybe a complete mile, around a few twists, up a few hills.

So here we were then. Going up the lift towards our floor. Upon entering the hospital my nerves began to kick in, a light agitation. I'm not sure if it was the fact that the appointment was looming, or whether it was just the hatred of hospitals. It could have been a combination of both I suppose. No matter, this was our floor. Disembarking from the lift we stepped out onto the floor, turning left and following the signs for the EDS clinic. At the end of the corridor we came to some double doors, locked at that. The only way in was via pressing the buzzer. Here we go then!

With a deep breath I reached my arm up and pressed the buzzer. Within a few seconds a voice came over the tannoy,

"Good morning" came the cheerful faceless voice of the lady variety.

"Good morning, it's David Malarky to see the genetics team."

With that there was a buzz, and pushing the big wooden fire doors back we entered!

2

Upon walking into the clinic we were immediately greeted by a courteous smile from behind the counter of the reception desk located directly in front of us. What immediately caught my attention was that the usual disinfectant hospital smell was not present here, nor was the coldness. There was a sort of warmth to the place. Yes the walls were painted in a standard magnolia, but looking over to the left from the reception and towards the waiting room, the walls had been plastered in drawings of pictures from all ages. There were crayon filled sheets of paper lining the walls like wallpaper. Pictures of sunshine, rainbows and smiley faces, stick children holding the hands of their stick parents. The waiting room was square shaped with rows of seats all around, but in the middle, tiny round tables sat with tiny plastic chairs in red and blue. Children's books sat on the tables, their colourfulness standing out against the dark wood surface. A giant toy box laden with toys. I felt a little out of place and old being here, but at the same time felt very much at ease.

Approaching the counter I reached into my pocket and unfolded my appointment letter. As soon as I got close I began to reach out to lay the paper on the counter.

"Good morning David, how are you doing today? You found us okay then?" came the woman's voice with a smile so wide.

I was a little taken aback that I didn't have to introduce myself. I had spent so much time going around these places and having to repeat myself time and time again it seemed like second nature to expect not to be known or why I was there.

"Good morning, I'm not too bad thanks, yeah we got here eventually, it wasn't that hard as we know Sheffield quite well."

"Ah that's okay then. You have come from Lincolnshire haven't you? Is this your dad?"

"Yeah we have, this is my father Howard."

"Nice to meet you Howard, I hope you are well."

"I'm not too bad thankyou, a little stiff from the drive." came my father's reply.

"Right, well you're a few minutes early for your appointment, looks like you made good time, so if you would like to take a seat in the waiting area and Hannah will be along shortly to go through what will be happening today if that's okay?"

"Yeah that's brilliant thanks." I said with a pleased smile!

A refreshing change this was. Not only did the lady know my name, she knew where I had come from, I had a feeling this appointment was going to have a slightly more personal touch rather than the feeling I was just another number waiting in line!

So take a seat we did. To my surprise the waiting room was empty, we had it all to ourselves. As soon as we had sat down I could hear the echoing of heeled shoes walking down the corridor in the distance. My father sat next to me flicking through a leaflet that had something to do with genetic testing, however my attention was focused up in front of me and to the right where the footsteps were getting closer. Then with graceful strides, a lady appeared from the corridor. Her dark ankle length skirt flowing behind as she moved along, her long dark hair down to the middle of her back, big wide eyes, small button nose. I could smell the scent of her perfume as she breezed past. As I'm not all that great with ages I didn't want to guess her age, but if I had to say I would have put her in her mid to late 20's.

My eyes followed her as she passed us, and she stopped at the reception desk where she briefly spoke to the smiley receptionist. Within a few seconds she had turned around and headed back, but instead of going back from where she came, she turned into the waiting area and straight towards us.

"Hello David."

"Please, call me Dave."

"Okay Dave, I'm Hannah, I just need to go through a couple of forms with you and ask for a signature or two, then I'd like to take you through to take your blood pressure, weight and height measurements if that's okay?" Her voice was soft and pleasing to the ear.

"Yeah that's all good thankyou."

From what I recall from my elusive memory, Hannah then went through a few forms and talked about how I would be seeing a doctor and a genetics counsellor, who would go through some of the things we previously talked about on the phone, then do a physical examination of myself. Taking the pen from her dainty hands, with fingernails painted a light pink in colour, I proceeded to sign on the dotted line.

"Thankyou very much, now if you would like to follow me."

"Of course I would."

Hannah led me into to small room opposite the waiting area. There wasn't a great deal in there apart from a few cupboards to the left, a standard hospital bed on the right, a set of scales and a height bar against the wall. After taking my weight and height I then sat down on the end of the bed, where she took my blood pressure.

135/82; that wasn't too bad compared to what it had been during the age of the elephants.

After all this was done it was once again back to the seats, where I planted myself next to my father. Hannah had said her goodbyes and had told us that it wouldn't be long before I would be going in. Today, I felt more relaxed than ever being here.

We weren't kept waiting long, within a few minutes another set of footsteps was heading down the corridor in our direction. This time a lady in her late 40's to early 50's, wearing thin framed round glasses and having short permed light brown hair came walking round the corner smiling across at us. Her name tag stuck out well, I could read her name was Rosemary and that she was the genetics counsellor.

"Good morning Dave."

She spoke with a familiar voice, I knew that voice!

"Good morning."

"I'm Rosemary and I'm the genetics counsellor you spoke to on the phone."

"Yes I thought I recognised the voice."

"Good morning Howard" directing her attention to my father.

"Good morning."

"If you'd both like to follow me, then we are ready for you just down the hall."

We arose from our seats and were led through the double doors to the corridor where she had come from. It was a long corridor with doors on either side going off to many different rooms. We didn't need to walk far though, as we entered the first door on the left. Walking in, Rosemary closed the door behind us.

Standing up to greet us again was another lady, somewhere around the same age as Rosemary, and from her name tag it turned out to be Dr Gazelle Banger. Where some of these names are coming from I really do not know! I can assure you, it's not myself, I would never do such things.

"Hello Dave, I'm Gazelle" as she reached out to shake my hand, "I believe you already know Rosemary from the phone interview?"

"Good morning, yes I remembered Rosemary's voice, it's nice to meet you both."

"And its nice to finally meet you, from the looks of it this is your father?"

"How did you guess?"

"There does seem to be a little resemblance."

"Thanks I think?"

Dr Gazelle went on to say, "Okay, so we know why we are all here. After speaking to you over the phone and going through your history and your father's history, it's pretty clear that there are underlying problems in your family. We believe it could be one of two things, one of them you had obviously heard about, Vascular Ehlers-Danlos Syndrome. What we would like to do is just go through a few details with yourself, then we shall give you a quick look over. Now with Vascular Ehlers-Danlos Syndrome it used to be that it was always diagnosed clinically via visual inspection and previous patient history, not in a lab. Only recently have blood tests become available to test for the mutated gene, so we should be able to give you an answer today, is that okay?"

"Yeah that's fine, I was kind of hoping it wouldn't get this far, but we are here so let's get it over with."

For the next ten or fifteen minutes we discussed all the information that we went through on the phone interview, going back through the family tree. My father at this point came to good use. He was able to fill in the blanks that I had left out, he was able to describe more of the situations that had arisen with himself and between us we got everything fully mapped out.

65

There was still of feeling of calmness in me. I'm not sure why it was, but I think it had a lot to do with the way I was being treated. It felt almost as if they were pleased to see me. I was made to feel very welcome, we were using first names and nothing was being rushed.

"Okay so now we have all the details and filled in some of the blanks, what I would like to do is take you into the examination room. Rosemary will take you through and give you a gown to put on, so if you could strip off for me."

With that being said I deep down really hoped that Gazelle didn't want me to strip off in some sort of dance routine, I'm quite certain that wouldn't have been appropriate.

Rosemary got to her feet and beckoned me to follow her through an open doorway off to the left of the room, which led to an examination room. She proceeded to hand me one of those blue faded chequered gowns which I just loved to wear. At least this time it wasn't cold in here. I took the gown and Rosemary left me to my own devices to get changed.

3

Slipping out of my clothes and into my gown I could hear muffled voices from behind the door. Rosemary and Gazelle were chatting away to my father, the topic of which I could not make out. The doors were of the heavy wood fire door type so not a lot really came through. As I stood there for a moment the muffled voices stopped and there came a knock at the door.

"Are you all fit Dave?" it was Gazelles voice, only

just making it into the room.

"Yep, I'm all ready for you."

With that Gazelle and Rosemary both came into the room, and Rosemary was holding a small digital camera. I could only assume this was for my portfolio pictures of this fine gown that I was now modelling.

"Okay what we need to do is just have a visual inspection around your body, then Rosemary is going to take a few pictures for the file."

With that Gazelle proceeded with her inspection. With pad in hand she began to closely look at my face, gently touching and inspecting my ears, moving down to my neck. As she did this she pulled the gown away from me slightly, checking my chest and moving round to my shoulders. I could see her placing ticks on the sheet of paper before her. If you remember back I did mention that in Vascular Ehlers-Danlos, one of the signs is visible veins. I could only assume this was what she was looking for.

Carrying on, Gazelle then took my hands in her hand, gently manipulating them, pushing the tips of my fingers slightly. She was slowly picking out the signs one by one. Looking at both sides of my hands she was checking my skin, then moving up to my elbows, she gently pulled my skin away from the bone. This one I didn't know, but turned out to be overly stretchy skin. Continuing down my body she came to my legs, where she slowly inspected the present bruises, the scar on my knee from when I was a child, and the veins that could easily be shown running their length.

"Alright Dave, if you could just bend over without bending your knees and touch your toes."

This I tried but fell a little bit short. It was quite evident that I wasn't as flexible as I had heard about, in the hypermobile sub category.

"Okay and now stand straight and push your knees

back as far as you can."

In doing this it appeared that my left knee was able to bend a little farther back than my right. I had recently started to get a lot of pain from my left knee, with no apparent cause for it when I'd had it checked out. Perhaps that was another one of those little things that could be accounted for.

"Okay, that's all we need. I'll just go write some notes while Rosemary takes the pictures."

With that Gazelle went back into the room where my father was still sat waiting.

"Right Dave, lets get this photo shoot started." said Rosemary with a little grin on her face.

"Would you like me to pose?"

"In a fashion I would actually yes."

"You best tell me where you want me then."

I even managed to let out a little chuckle.

What was to follow made me feel like a real model, or not, as the case may be. The hospital gown wasn't exactly flattering my figure. Rosemary took pictures of my hands, chest, back, neck, legs, pretty much everything that Gazelle had just gone over. These pictures would be going in my file to keep for reference in the future, I believed. Either that or I'd one day stumble across myself in a copy of "Hospital Gown Weekly"!

After she was finished Rosemary went back into the room. The visual examination was over. It had been fun being inspected from top to toe, but it was now time to get myself dressed. As I did this, there were no muffled voices this time, only silence back in the room beyond, where my father, Rosemary and Gazelle were now waiting.

Fully clothed once again I took myself back to my seat next to my father. Rosemary sat in front of me slightly to my left, and Gazelle sat directly in front of me. She was leant over the desk slightly, just finishing off filling out the form. For a moment there was silence. The atmosphere seemed to have changed a little. I still felt comfortable, however as I was looking round the room I caught Rosemary's gaze, and there was something in her eyes, a slight look of sadness maybe. With that, the silence was broken as Gazelle sat back up and put her pen down, looking at me she began to talk.

"Right sorry about that Dave, I just had to finish filling that in. As I said previously, Vascular Ehlers-Danlos Syndrome was always diagnosed clinically. There are a few visual signs we look for, big eyes, thin nose, thin lips, small chin, lobeless ears. We also look at the visibility of the veins in your skin, flexibility on the extremities, i.e. fingers. And as you know we also go from past history of yourself and relatives that may have had problems."

She paused for a second as if composing her thoughts, a delicacy now entered her voice that wasn't there before. Her eyes had lost that glint of happiness and were instead filled with a sympathetic look.

"Taking all this into consideration I would have to say that yes, you do have Vascular Ehlers-Danlos Syndrome."

There was silence all round. Not a single sound could be heard, not even the ticking of a clock. Those last words she said seemed to disappear off into nothing, spoken but not heard.

Still silence.

My head moved around to the right, my father's eyes were transfixed on the ground. I looked back towards Gazelle and then over to Rosemary. They were just sat there watching me, still, not speaking, just full of deep meaningful looks. I suppose if you think about it, this couldn't have been easy for them. They had probably done this sort of thing a hundred times, confirming someone's worst fears, but I should imagine everyone reacts differently. Maybe some people break down and cry, maybe some people argue that they can't be right. Myself, I didn't feel anything. It had just been confirmed that I was right, what I had stumbled on, the worst case, the rarest thing anyone could ever think of, and it was right. But nothing, there was no great emotion inside of me, no welling of the eyes, no arguments, just nothing.

To me it felt like time had slowed down. Nobody was saying anything at all, not until I saw Rosemary's hand come up, and she placed it on my knee.

"Are you ok Dave?"

"Yeah I'm fine."

"It's okay if you want to cry."

I can honestly say I felt no different whatsoever. I wasn't smiling, I wasn't angry, nor was I upset. Perhaps it was shock, I can't really be sure. Gravity wasn't weighing down on me.

So as the sombre moment had gone on way too long I looked at them both and blurted out,

"So what now?"

"One step at a time" came Gazelle's reply. "As I said, although Vascular Ehlers-Danlos Syndrome had always been clinically diagnosed, we can do a blood test to identify the mutation in the gene. Once we get the results back we will be able to diagnose family members. Your father, your sister, your brother and your son will all need testing, but first we would have to test your blood. That takes about eight weeks."

With that said, in the back of my mind something registered a little. This wasn't just about me any more, this no longer affected just me. Now they were bringing the rest of the family into it, my brother, my sister … my son. My son. Not a chance, that couldn't be. I'm sure if they did the blood test then they would find that they wouldn't be right. They must have made a mistake.

"Okay then yes, let's do the blood test. It could still come back negative right?"

"Well there is a slim chance, but with regards to everything we have looked we are pretty certain. do you understand what this means?" came Rosemary.

"Yes pretty much, you're saying I have a life threatening condition that has no cure and can strike at any time. Surely there is something we can do right?"

"For now it's best to wait for the blood tests. Try not to lift anything heavy or strain yourself too much, and try to keep your blood pressure low, this is important. When we get the blood tests results back, we will ring you to see you again, then we will organise an appointment with a cardiologist. You will have to have an MRI to check the arteries for aneurysms and will be monitored yearly. Any questions you have in the meantime you can always ring us. Even if its just to talk we are still here for you."

There were now hundreds of questions whizzing round my head. What about this, what about that, what if, what if??? The one thing I hung onto was the fact they wanted to do the blood test. If they wanted to do this then surely they could be wrong? Surely this would mean there was a possibility it might come back negative? Even if it was a slim chance, look how slim the chance was of me stumbling onto this. There was still time, I wouldn't give up hope just yet that this was the demon that stood before us, the demon that was inside of us trying to break us down. Not this.

"Okay let's do the blood test then and see what happens. One step at a time right?" I replied.

"Yes, that's the way to do it. Rosemary will take you in the other room and take a blood sample whilst I finish off writing the notes."

Rosemary got up from her chair and took me back through to the examination room. She had quite a hard time managing to get any blood out of me. This was no different to anyone else though. The simplest task of drawing blood from me seemed to be like getting blood from a stone. As we walked back down the corridor past the waiting room and towards the big wooden doors to exit the clinic, Rosemary continued to talk to me. What she seemed to be saying was going in one ear and out the other, but she was trying to console me, reassure me. She was trying to let me know that if I needed anything, they were only a phone call away and that I shouldn't hesitate to ring. Of course I wouldn't do this, why on earth would I want to phone up this stranger, as nice and friendly as she was, and talk about my inner feelings. No, I would be fine!

The ride home was pretty quiet apart from the background music of the radio. I wasn't really thinking of anything at all. My mind seemed to have drifted off into a place of nothingness. Again there were no feelings there, I just felt numb and kind of empty. I was in my own little world, cars whizzing by, the day had been long and I just wanted to get back to the comfort of my own home. No more talking about it, no more thinking about it.

4

For a moment I would like to take you away from the story, not for long mind, as I'm sure you're very eager to learn more of the events. I'm sure you are waiting with great anticipation for these next eight weeks to pass for the results. I was too. However I have taken a few days off writing this. The main reason being my fingers have been struggling to type a little. My head has been struggling to process a little. When I started to type this I perhaps underestimated the task at hand. I am quite handy with a keyboard, I build my own computers and spend a lot of time using them, I just didn't realise that I would be typing so much.

Anyway, whilst I was having this little break I have been looking around the mystical internet at all manner of things. There is something that I would like to share with you. It does seem relevant to the story that is now unfolding and perhaps now is a good time to incorporate it into the book. If I'm honest, looking back over past events I can see the logic behind it. What is it you ask? Well, its this:

DABDA

No I haven't made up a random word, well not this time anyway. Its an acronym. Some of you may have come across this before. It's not something I had come across, but as I read about it, it seemed to make a lot of sense. It seemed to fit in with the next set of events that had now begun to kick off.

For those of you that have not come across this before I will briefly explain. DABDA is a hypothesis that was introduced by Elisabeth Kubler-Ross in 1969 when she wrote a book on death and dying, which was inspired by her work with terminally ill patients. It describes the five stages of grief that people are often found to go through when faced with a life threatening/altering event. Now this doesn't always apply to everyone, and not necessarily in this order, but those stages are:

1) Denial
2) Anger
3) Bargaining
4) Depression
5) Acceptance

As I now look back, with a clearer head than I had a few weeks ago, I can see where this all fits in with everything I have experienced. All of these steps feature at some point in this journey I seem to have encountered, and it makes sense of some of the actions that I have taken. If you try to remember DABDA in the back of your mind while we carry on, you may also see these stages come into play, and maybe you will even agree with me. But anyway, shall we ride the train further down the line? … Yes lets!

5

The next eight weeks if I'm completely honest, are still a bit of a blur. Time did go by very slowly. I tried to carry on as normal as possible. As far as I was concerned, although I had been clinically diagnosed, it still wasn't real. Even though this was a solid basis for being diagnosed I didn't really believe it and it didn't hold a lot of weight for me. After all, I'd only been looked over by a couple of people that I had never seen before, so surely they couldn't just tell by looking at me. The blood test result would be the only result I would trust in. In the meantime I would try not to think about it.

As the days turned into weeks I thought I was doing alright. My curiosity was mostly kept at bay. Of course in the back of my mind though it was always eating away at me. Like a guinea pig constantly gnawing away. I use the animal guinea pig as my sister has a great love for these furry creatures. I can just imagine their little mouths moving around and around chewing and gnawing. When I was occupied during the day, everything went well. It was the nights that were the hardest. I remember lying in bed, questions going around and around, sending me dizzy. If only the brain would had an off switch. There were many nights I would lie awake until three or maybe four in the morning, sometimes just staring into the darkness, sometimes bombarding myself with different thoughts.

I had told myself that I wasn't going to look into anything else at this moment in time. But this was impossible. There were a few times that I would once again search on the internet. It was here I discovered the first YouTube video. As I previously stated, there isn't a lot to find about Vascular Ehlers-Danlos out there, and most of what you do find, you'd rather have not have found it. But I think human nature makes us look.

The first video I came across was the story of a young couple. It was only a short video, but the impact was hard. It told the story of a young couple and of the male who had had a lifetime of unusual medical complications but he was always active and had a passion for life. It told of how his splenic artery ruptured in his sleep, nearly taking away his life. A few months later it would turn out that he was diagnosed with Vascular Ehlers-Danlos. A month later he was found to have aneurysms on his iliac arteries and taken into ICU. Whilst this was going on, his other half had been pregnant and was about to give birth to his child. She gave birth to their child while he was in intensive care and took the baby to meet him in his hospital bed. A few weeks later, he died from a ruptured abdominal aortic aneurysm. He was 27 years of age. Another two weeks later and it was confirmed that their son also had Vascular Ehlers-Danlos Syndrome. The video wasn't one to gain sympathy, yes it was a heartbreaking story, but it was about the fight to raise awareness to try and gain the support to get much needed research.

This, in my mind, would only reinforce the fact that

the blood test would hopefully come back negative. Everything was feeling kind of surreal, like one of those afternoon made for TV medical dramas you come across and can't help but watch sometimes. Things like this didn't happen in real life, not to me anyway.

It was getting near to the end of the eight weeks and finally a phone call came from Sheffield. They wanted to make another appointment to see me again in a couple of weeks. It would turn out to be August 22nd 2013. This date, I wouldn't be forgetting, not only because of the appointment, but another event miles away from myself was taking place.

6

The 22nd soon came around. Again we would be setting off on another journey to the land of Yorkshire to find out the fate of what lay ahead. This time, my mother would come along for the ride as well as my father. With her working in a school it meant that she was off for the six weeks holidays. It was nearly like a summer day trip out, only we forgot to pack a picnic! That's okay though, we would be once again be whizzing into that halfway McDonalds stop.

Arriving at the EDS clinic, we were again greeted with smiling faces. That pleasurable feeling of being known not as a number but as an actual person. It was kind of funny how I enjoyed going there. But when you have been tossed from pillar to post, when you have had to wait for people to go through your notes, when you have had to explain the situation over and over again to someone that hasn't got a clue as why you are in front of them, it really is nice to be known. Unfortunately there was no Hannah this morning. This was a shame I thought to myself. It would have been nice to start the day on that vision, however we had been through all the measuring and weighing previously and it wasn't needed this time around, more important matters were at hand.

There was no waiting around in the waiting room this time. Instead we walked straight towards the reception desk and as soon as we did Rosemary was gracefully gliding down the corridor to meet us. She must have had a tip off that we had arrived when we pressed the buzzer to the clinic doors. Either that or she wasn't telling us something, psychic abilities? Hmm well I guess anything is possible right? There are some strange occurrences in this world, so perhaps Rosemary was hiding this little fact.

"Good morning David, good morning Mum and Dad, its Gertrude isn't it? We haven't met before, I'm Rosemary."

"Good morning. Yes that's right it's Gertrude, it's nice to meet you." came my mother's reply.

With this Rosemary raised her arm around my shoulder and beckoned us to follow her.

"So how have you been feeling Dave?"

"I've not been too bad thanks, just been cracking on as usual. Work work and more work."

"That's good to hear, it's nice to see you back and smiling."

As we walked down the corridor towards that same room we carried on back and forth with a little small talk to ease the nerves, which I guess were showing a little. As we went into the room, Dr Gazelle Banger was already there, ready and waiting with my notes out. I was beginning to feel a little eager and just wanted to get the results. It had been a long eight weeks and finally I just wanted to know one way or another. Although I tried my hardest to put it to the back of my mind, the strain had been taking it's toll. Rosemary went on to introduce my mother to Gazelle, then we established that everyone was well and we were ready to begin.

"Right David."

Gazelle's voice was soft, quiet, my ears had to turn slightly to hear her.

"As you know, we met here eight weeks ago and clinically diagnosed you via a physical exam with Vascular Ehlers-Danlos Syndrome. We then sent your blood away for further testing to identify the mutated gene. We now have the results back for you."

As I cleared my throat and I let out a whimper of "Okay" I sounded like some sort of wounded dog. My throat had suddenly become very dry. The heat in the room had started to make me sweat a little. I could feel my eyes roaming around the room not exactly sure where to look. Rosemary's eyes were cast upon me. Gazelle's eyes were cast upon me. Just beyond Gazelle there was a window and across from us was another part of the building. For some reason I started to count the bricks on the wall. Why was I doing that? I was supposed to be listening, after all this was a little important.

"When the blood is being tested we are looking for a ..."

And I'm back in the room. For a moment I had completely drifted off into my own little world, counting those bricks one at a time. Concentrate man!

".. a mutation in the COL3A1 gene. The blood test has come back and verified that you have this mutation, meaning that it confirms the clinical diagnosis of Vascular Ehlers-Danlos Syndrome."

And that was it. The silence that had come once before filled the room, nothing, no ticking of a clock, just pure silence. Five people sat in this room, stillness, silence. My eyes were transfixed on the window, the bricks, counting, fast, faster, going down the line wanting to count everything single last brick, 25, 30, 40. My mind was working overtime to count all those red worn bricks before anybody could break the silence, 55, 60. I couldn't think of anything else, I had Vascular Ehlers-Danlos, I had this random rare life threatening condition that had caused so many problems with in my family for years and years. Silently striking us, trying to take us down one by one, hiding inside us like an alien waiting to rip out of our chests. It was real, it was my family's demon. It was haunting us … but the bricks, 75, 80, just counting the bricks.

"David?"

"David … are you okay?"

I heard Rosemary's voice but it didn't register.

"Are you okay, David?" again the voice came softly.

Good question. Was I okay? I didn't really know. I was okay, but I wasn't okay. In a moment I'm sure I would wake and it would all be a distant nightmare. But I didn't. The past events had led me along this path and here we sat in this room, being told something that nobody should hear. You think you are prepared to hear something like this, you're not, how can you be? Nothing can prepare you for anything like this. Nothing has changed, its been plaguing our family for years, but everything has changed. We know its name, we know it's power. Its a stone cold killer, and now it had just become real.

"Yeah I'm fine, I think." I finally replied after taking a deep breath and recomposing myself.

"So that's it then, it is definitely this Vascular Ehlers-Danlos Syndrome?"

"Yes, I'm afraid so." came Gazelle's almost inaudible reply.

"So I was right?"

"Yes you were."

"Well to be honest I was hoping to be laughed out of here a long time ago. I didn't think for a minute that it would actually get this far, I kinda wish it hadn't."

"With something like this it is better to know, although we can't do a lot. As you know there is no miracle cure and not a lot is known, but if you know about it then you can have everything in place that will help you if complications do occur."

"I suppose you're right in that respect! So what can we do? What can I do? What's next?"

There now seemed to be a lot of questions building up in the back of my head all wanting to come out in a tangled mess. My mother and father were remaining pretty silent. I supposed they were taking it all in, which was perhaps a good thing, as I knew most of what I was going to be told would be going straight in one ear and out the other.

For a moment there was silence again, as if Gazelle was coming up with some great battle plan, some way of slaying the demon maybe? Then Rosemary looked across to my mother and father.

"Before we go on, Mum and Dad, are you both okay? Is there anything you want to ask?"

My mother looked back at Rosemary, her eyes seemed a little wide, I could see she was fighting off the water droplets that were trying to break free from her eyes and she replied softly with a little upturn in her mouth trying to give off a smile.

"Yeah we're okay, just a little taken aback. As David said, we were hoping in the back of our minds that the tests would come back negative. It all feels a little surreal."

"It's not an easy thing to process and it will take time, if you have any questions at all, even after the appointment you can ring us any time."

The atmosphere was terrible. Fake smiles, quiet voices. It felt like somewhere inside a little piece of me had died. Had it? We had been through a lot but this felt different, this was me, my father had been in the same position when he was diagnosed with Hypertrophic Cardiomyopathy. He must have had similar sorts of words said to him, how did he react, what did they say? How do you process something like this? Is my life ever going to be the same again? How was my mother feeling, she was in the room when this happened to my dad, and here she is again going through the same thing with me. Thoughts, many, many thoughts whizzing around inside, so many questions. Making sense of it all was bordering on the lines of impossible. Even though I have grown up around this type of thing, I never actually thought for one minute that the day would come when I would be sat in a room being told this life changing news. It happens in movies all the time, and to other people around you, but it's never going to happen to you, or so I thought anyway. I guess I was a little wrong on that one eh!

Dr Gazelle began to speak again.

"Okay what you can do yourself is to avoid any heavy lifting, a little exercise can be good, either walking, swimming, but nothing that is high impact like weights or running. Your blood pressure needs to be monitored and kept low, which I know you're taking tablets for anyway so we are on the right track there. Apart from that we will scan your arteries once a year checking for aneurysms. I will make you an appointment to see our specialist cardiologist here in Sheffield who will look after you and monitor you."

"Okay, that's good, so what else, is there a list of do's and don'ts?

"Well with Vascular Ehlers-Danlos its different for everybody. You have to find a balance between living and not living. The important thing is to be careful, but don't lock yourself away from the world. You still have to try and live as normal life as you can. We have an information pack for you which explains Vascular Ehlers-Danlos Syndrome, it contains a copy of a medical alert information sheet, and also a leaflet regarding medi alerts. We would advise that you get a medi alert bracelet and wear it at all times. If you have a complication and need to go to hospital then this will tell the doctors about your condition and will outline the importance, as not many people will really know about it."

Gazelle picked up a white folder with Ehlers-Danlos Syndrome National Diagnostic Service emblazoned across the front of it. I reached out for it and took it out of her hands. Upon opening it, I discovered inside the medical alert information, a little leaflet about Vascular Ehlers-Danlos and the medical alert pamphlet. Attached to the folder was a business card with Rosemary's number and title, "genetic counsellor" on it. I guess this was here for when I needed to talk about my deep dark inner feelings. I'm Dave Malarky. Of course I wouldn't need to do that!

"With Ehlers-Danlos Syndrome being a genetic hereditary syndrome it would also be very important to test other family members. It is important to get your son tested, your sister and perhaps dad."

Rosemary's words hit me like a punch to the gut.

Gordon, no not Gordon, that wouldn't be fair, he's only ten. The world can be a nasty place, but it's not that nasty surely!

"Testing Gordon is something I would have to speak to his mum about. I mean if nothing can really be done, do we really need to? It's going to change his life. He plays football, he loves football, I can't take things like that away from him, he's just a kid!"

I could feel a little anger welling up at the thought of

this.

"Although nothing solid can be done, it would be best to put him in the best possible position to be cared for. Do you think he has any symptoms?"

"I don't know, a few maybe. He usually has bruises, but he's a boy, an active boy. Boys play rough so he will always have bruises.." I let out a deep sigh, "the tips of his fingers bend back like mine, and he does look similar to how I did when I was his age."

My mother suddenly burst to life, "Yes, he's the spitting image of David when he was that age."

For another moment there was silence. That cold eerie silence that made the hair on the back of your neck stand to attention. I now didn't like where this was going. Not only had I been diagnosed, but now it was going after more people. None of this seemed right, none of it seemed fair.

"It would be an idea to get him tested. There is a 50/50 chance that it has been passed on, but like you say, he is a boy and young boys play rough so it's very hard to tell with children. But there would be great benefit to knowing and it will give him a greater chance for the future. Obviously you will have to discuss that with his mother, but all you need to do if you decide to go ahead is get a referral from his local GP. It's quite straightforward, if you just explain the situation and give them our details, the same for any family member who wants to be diagnosed, including Franny."

Rosemary now turned her gaze upon Howard, my father, who had remained quite silent throughout the whole experience, well, apart from the odd grunt and nod here and there.

"Now Howard, It would be a good idea to start off with you. It does sound like it stems from further back in the family, but if we could test yourself then we can rule that out and no-one else would need testing. Would you be okay with that?"

"To be honest it really makes no difference to me, I've always had problems anyway and I'm still here, but yes if it helps we can do that."

Finally my father came into play, unfazed by the possibility that he could be diagnosed. But then he was right, it wouldn't really make any difference to him, as he has known these bizarre problems all his life.

"If you don't mind then, we can take you into the back room and do the physical exam like we did on David last time and then take some blood to be sent away. Would that be okay?"

"Yeah that's fine, go for it."

Dr Gazelle Banger and Rosemary took my father through to the examination room that I had been in previously. They were obviously going through the exact same process they had gone through with me eight weeks previously. In the meantime, my mother and myself were left to our own thoughts. Thoughts of which I cannot really remember. So much was unfolding on this day. Not only had I just been diagnosed we were now moving forward to talk about other family members. Over the last two years everything had gone so slow. Time for a while had seemed to be standing still, a road that was so long and twisty leading us here. Now we were here, now I had been diagnosed. It was like someone had suddenly pressed the fast forward button. It seemed like an age ago that I had done a little research, stumbled across this rare random evilness, and now here we were making it all so real. From frame advance to fast forward in one fell swoop. If you ever had a VCR, then you will now what I'm talking about there. If you didn't, then you're just a youngster, Google it!

It didn't take long, within five or ten minutes, maybe more maybe less, in this room time didn't really exist or have any meaning, my father reappeared and came to sit between my mother and myself. He was followed in by Gazelle and Rosemary who both sat down.

"Ok Howard" came Gazelle's voice, "after looking at you it is quite clear that you also share very similar features to Dave, and a lot of the criteria for a clinical diagnosis of Vascular Ehlers-Danlos. I'm sure this hasn't come as any surprise to yourself."

"Not really no, but it doesn't really make any difference to me."

Rosemary took a sorrowful glance at myself, then my mother, and then turned her focus back to my father.

"In a way this is a good thing, as now we know to check the rest of the family. We can do a blood test on yourself Howard, which shouldn't take as long to come back as Dave's, as we already know the mutation we are looking for. At least if we know about it, and if we find other family members with it, then we can get the correct care system in place to give everyone the best possible chance against it."

"So you will be wanting some of my blood aswell then? You can take as much as you want, I'm quite used to being prodded and poked now."

My head had now become a little dazed. I felt like I was in some kind of half awake half asleep dream state. Not really knowing what was real and what was not. A fog had swirled its way into my brain, clouding my vision, wrapping its self around my thoughts. I knew what was going on, but I couldn't grasp the reality of it all. Here we sat, in this room, five people, discussing the dark demon that flows through us. Something that had been with us all our lives, hiding in the shadows silently, waiting, striking out at us, causing pain and despair throughout generations of our family.

Now we know you demon, now you have a face. Fear, confusion, chaos. You are my one true enemy. I can't run from you, I can't hide from you, for you lie within the confines of my very own body.

CHAPTER 4
MORE THAN MEETS THE EYE

I wanted that day to end. But it wasn't quite over yet. There was yet another task at hand. One that I really didn't want to carry out on that day as the mind was still shrouded in the fog. However the way it played out, there were events that had to take place.

I don't like seriousness, too much seriousness makes you frown, gives you wrinkles. I like to laugh and have a joke, to mess around and have a little fun. But lately seriousness seemed to have taken over. It makes you tired, it makes you grow up. Even now I'm still not that sure I want to grow up. Inside of me there is still my younger self. I still like to be silly, pull faces, make people jump, make crazy ass videos on my phone to lighten up the seriousness of life. I don't know about you, but when I was younger I always wondered what it would be like to be an adult, to go to work everyday, have my own house, own family, I always dreamed of being older than I was. Now, well I would love to go back to being small again. Go back to school, hang out with my school mates, have endless days of fun not really having anything of great importance to worry about. It was so much safer back then. None of this seriousness business!

So anyway, back to the story of events at hand. I do hope you're keeping up. I may have to go back and tidy my story a little for it all to makes sense, although maybe not, as Vascular Ehlers Danlos is one of those things in this world that doesn't make sense. Any way you look at it, it never will.

Onwards we go then. We had left the hospital and were on our way home. I had taken to the back seat and let my mother handle the ride of the superb old Ford Focus I had picked up a few months ago. All I wanted to do was sit in the back, look out the window and stroke my beard whilst contemplating the events of the day. I can honestly say that I didn't really know what I was actually feeling within myself. What I can remember is that my thoughts drifted towards my son, Gordon.

He was a good kid, a great kid. He was full of life, and didn't deserve to have this legacy thrust upon him. They wanted to test him, but what were the benefits in this. If he had it, it would change his life. Would he have to stop playing football? Would we have to wrap him up in bubble wrap in fear of anything happening? Why? Why put this on someone so young? Children are meant to play, children are meant to live without fear, without seriousness. I didn't want to have brought this onto my child. Would we really want to know?

But in reality, it was too late for that. The path had been chosen, what else was there to do. If he wasn't tested, there would always be that doubt in the back of the mind. Yes if it was positive it would change his life, but at least it would give him a fighting chance for the future. In my mind I guess the answer was sort of clear, he did need to be tested, but would his mother see it that way.

My phone was in my pocket. Now was perhaps not the best of times to do this, but I reached for it. I decided I had to text his mother. It was to be a simple text stating that I needed to speak to her, to set a time to go round and explain the situation without Gordon there. Together we would have to come to a decision about whether or not he should be tested. Luckily I have an amicable relationship with his mother. We had split a long time ago when Gordon was only 18 months old. At first, things were a little hairy but over the years we have always managed to put our differences aside and put Gordon first. Whilst we aren't exactly what I would call friends, we can talk to each other, so this would make it a little easier. I didn't want to do it on this day as things were still unclear and I needed a little time to get my head around everything that was unfolding. However after sending a couple of texts back and forth, I spoke to his mother on the phone. It turned out this evening was the time to do it.

We had barely got home, and had a lovely cup of tea, which I have to admit I did slurp a little. I like to slurp my tea at my Mum and Dad's house. I say it enables you to get a little more flavour out, but in reality I do it because it winds my sister Franny up. She glares at me, and it makes me chuckle! Sorry Franny, I am a very bad person! My mother does make a nice cup of tea though. Over the years she has mastered the art of it, although sometimes she does forget to add my sugar. I like two sugars, not one but two, definitely not without any at all. I need to something to sweeten me up!

After speaking to mother dearest, she decided that she would come with me. This obviously wasn't going to be the easiest of conversations. I would have to explain exactly what Vascular Ehlers-Danlos was in simple terms to Gordon's mother, what the implications of it are, how it was the cause of my dissection, but at the same time I didn't really want her to be scared. The thought that Gordon had a 50/50 chance of having it was one of the most scary thoughts I've ever had. For myself I could handle it, or at least I thought I could, but for Gordon it was a different ball game entirely, and one that struck up a great fear inside of me.

Gordon lives a few towns away from myself. So another little drive was in order. It wasn't all that far away, around about a forty-five minute drive. Years ago I used to live there with Gordon's mother in a three bedroomed mid-terraced house. It wasn't too bad a place to live, a reasonably sized port town. I wasn't the keenest on it, but at the time house prices over there were cheaper than they were in my home town, so that's where I bought my first house. The drive over there this time round seemed to take forever. I was rehearsing in my head what I was going to say, over and over again. I had the folder with me that I had been given in Sheffield by Gazelle and Rosemary. I was sure the medical alert sheet within would help me with the task.

Upon arrival we pulled up outside of Sandy's house; Sandy being Gordon's mother, which I have obviously neglected to tell you yet. I do apologise for this. Going to the door of the end terraced house in this quiet cul de sac, I had barely raised my hands to knock when the door opened revealing Sandy standing there with a look of concern on her face. Obviously she wanted to know what was going on that was so important. Sandy had known about the problems I had had over the past couple of years, she knew of all the problems, the complications and the pain that my father had been going through for the past thirty years. Like the rest of us though, we thought his problems were down to the Hypertrophic Cardiomyopathy, and since we had been tested for this, didn't think that my problems were remotely related to his.

"Hi, come in. Would you like a drink, tea coffee?" There was an air of concern in her voice.

"Yeah can I have a tea please, two sugars, it's been a long day." my reply came.

"I'm okay thanks, I'm all tea'd out for the day." said my mother.

As Sandy went through to the kitchen to put the kettle down we sat on the sofa. The house wasn't the biggest of houses but was quite cosy. The front door let you straight into what was a sort of open plan living room, filled with two seater sofas laid out in an L-shape, with a small passageway between which led you back to the stair area. The stairs in this place were awesome. They were shiny polished wood and sat behind the sofa to the right, and as you walked up them they would twist round, meaning that you had a small under stair area behind the sofa, where the computer desk snuggled.

With the clinking of cups, Sandy emerged back through the archway and into the living room from the kitchen, steam coming out of the freshly brewed tea.

In a soft and slightly quivering voice I began to speak.

"I've been to see some specialists in a Childrens Hospital today, and got some results back from some blood tests that I've had done." As the words came out I was clutching the information folder that I had been given tightly in my hand.

"The Childrens Hospital, aren't you a little old for going there now?" Sandy's reply came across a little like she was taking the mick, but had an edge of curiosity.

"Yeah I guess I am a little, but it's where the genetics team are based."

"Okay what's the genetics team?"

"They are the guys that have diagnosed me. They deal with hereditary conditions and they have given me a diagnosis. The reason I need to speak to you is that there is a 50/50 chance that I could have passed it onto Gordon, so we need to discuss whether we get him tested or not!"

"Okay well what have they said? What is it that you have been diagnosed with?" Sandy's eyebrows raised a little as the question popped out.

"You won't have heard of it but it is something called

Vascular Ehlers-Danlos Syndrome."

"Er .. no, not heard of that one, what is it it?" She raised a little smile not having a clue what I was talking about.

"In a nutshell it's a life threatening condition which means we have mutated genes affecting the collagen. Collagen is like the foundation to a house. It holds us together like a glue, however our glue is faulty which means it can lead to complications throughout our bodies. Arteries and veins can tear, hollow organs can rupture and a lot of other things can randomly happen."

I was quite amazed at the way I was calmly trying to explain, but again this all still felt like a movie and didn't seem real in the slightest, maybe I was just dreaming!

"This leaflet perhaps explains it a little better than I can." I arose slightly from my seat and reached over to give Sandy the information pack that I was still clutching tightly.

Sandy reached out and took it from my hands, slowly removing the medical alert sheet from the folder.

"So what are they going to do?"

"To be honest with you, there is nothing they can do. There is no cure and very little is known about it. All I've been told to do is keep my blood pressure low, avoid doing anything too physical, I can walk and go swimming."

"What do you mean nothing? There must be something you can take?" Her eyes were now wandering down the medical alert sheet.

"I can take blood pressure tablets, and they will scan my body for aneurysms once a year, but apart from that, problems will be treated as they arise."

For a moment there was silence, as Sandy took in what she was reading. I could see a glint her her eyes from where she was trying to hold back the droplets of water that were forming.

"This is horrible. They can't operate on you?"

"Well they can but only with special vascular surgeons present and if it's a life threatening situation where my chances of survival are low anyway. Because the arteries are weak, it can cause more problems."

"So this is what caused your problems a couple of years ago?"

"Yes, not only that, it looks like it has caused all my Dad's problems over the years, and also the early death of my grandma and her mother before that. It seems to have been in the family for years. Dad was clinically diagnosed with it today and has had his blood sent off as well for confirmation."

"Well why didn't they find it earlier? Howard hasn't been well for years, I thought it was the HCM?"

Sandy was looking a little overwhelmed, I guess she had always thought I had perhaps dramatised things a little and wasn't expecting anything like this.

"Because it's so rare and not many people know about it. Of all the types, vascular is one of the rarest, it apparently affects around 1 in 250,000. I think a rare disease is classed as 1 in 2,500."

"Yeah but surely someone he has seen will have heard of it? He's seen loads of specialists?"

"He has, but they haven't looked at the overall bigger picture and put the pieces together. When I had my dissection I came across this EDS on the internet, obviously knowing my dad's problems, my family history and then my problems, I thought the pieces all seemed to fit and took my findings to my doctor, who agreed and pointed us in the right direction."

"Well this is crazy. Trust you lot to have something this rare."

I think a little wit was meant with that but it seemed to flow off in a totally different direction.

"Well if we could have chosen then I could think of

many more things that we would rather have than this, but the main reason I've told you is because we need to make a decision about Gordon. He can be tested with a simple blood test, but with them not being able to do anything, the question is do we get him tested? I think we should, as if he does have it, then at least we can have things in place to give him the best chance. We could also help him avoid anything that will make things worse. On the other hand it will change his life, but then also if we don't we will always have that nagging feeling in the back of our minds. Going off some of the symptoms I think he will be okay, but there's always that doubt."

Sandy's reply came quick.

"I think we should, we can't not. It's horrible but we need to know."

"Yep I think we do too, I'm glad you agree."

"So how do we do it then? Do we ring them up?"

"No, they only take referrals from doctors, what you will have to do is phone up the doctor, or go and see them, explain the situation about my diagnosis and ask them to write Gordon a referral letter to the EDS clinic in Sheffield. You shouldn't have any problems but if you do, then one of the ladies, Rosemary will be able to ring and speak to the doctor."

"Okay well I'll give them a ring now then."

What a day this was turning out to be. I felt like I was being swept up by a whirlwind with no control of the events that were now unfolding. I had gone from waiting, waiting and more waiting, to being diagnosed, my father being clinically diagnosed and now getting things in place for Gordon to be tested. There was no time for reality to really sink in. Everything had been put onto fast forward, and everything was happening with such urgency. Now. Not tomorrow, not next week. But now, no breathing space, no time to think.

My mother and I sat around quietly while Sandy was on the phone to the doctors. She left a message for the doctor to ring her back. I was hoping that they would just and do the letter as I didn't want Gordon to have to sit there and hear any more than was necessary. He was only ten years old, so he didn't need to know all of the ins and outs. It would be much better if the doctor could just refer him without wanting to see him. Which would also bring us to the next step of having to explain why he needed a blood test.

The phone went down and Sandy came to join us back in the front room.

"We need to tell Gordon something about why he is having a blood test. He's round at my mum's, so if you have time shall we go round there and talk to him?"

"To be honest I really don't feel like it today, I pick him up tomorrow night for the weekend so I'd like to let things sink in, as at the minute my head is all over the place, besides that will give me chance to work out a way of explaining it to him without upsetting him too much."

"I really think you should do it now. If I go and get him, he will know something is up. I hadn't said you were coming over, but he will just know something is wrong, I won't be able to hide it from him and will have to say something. At least if you are here then he will see you are okay. Well sort of okay, and he won't worry so much."

Her view was valid I guess, but bloody hell this was all going so fast. Talk about a roller coaster ride, I wanted to get off!

My mother chipped in. "I think it would be best for you to tell him as well, you don't have to go into all the details but at least if he sees you then it will be a little better!"

"Grrr … okay."

I let out a little unamused growl, but I guess they were both right. It did make sense but it would just have been nice to sleep on it. I really didn't know what I was going to say. How do you explain something so serious to a ten year old without upsetting him? And then telling him that he needs a test too to make sure he is okay. Madness, complete madness. But this was the situation so it had to be dealt with!

2

A short drive away and there we were. At Gordon's other grandparents house. He had no idea that I was coming, and I had no idea what I was going to tell him. I had been trying to think about what I was going to say in the ten minute drive it took to get there. In reality, nothing came to light, not a thing. This is why I didn't want to go there that evening. I would have liked a little time to prepare for it. Mind you given another twenty four hours, would I still be able to come up with anything? Really, what do you say? How do you explain? If only life was uncomplicated, but then I guess it would be boring as there would be no challenges before us. What's life without a good challenge eh! A spanner in the works keeps our minds sharp, keeps us on our toes and agile.

The front door opened straight into the living room, and seated there were Roger and Mary. In the years that I had been with Sandy, Roger and Mary had been like a second set of parents to me. They weren't the usual in laws that you can't stand being around, they were family. We had shared many ups and downs and used to be very close. We even lived just one street away from them at one point. On a weekend I would spend many an evening sat with Roger sinking down Bacardi and cokes, whilst playing "Bomber Man" on the PlayStation. Sometimes we even went shopping together and played "Bomber Man" around the store, but that's another story.

As I walked in I saw both their faces change into a look of surprise, curiousness as to why I had suddenly turned up. Gordon wasn't in the front room but was upstairs playing on the computer in the bedroom. If this was the reaction I got from them as I walked through the door, I knew he would immediately be questioning why I was there. Hello's were said and the offer of tea or coffee was placed, but politely refused, a feeling of sickness had entered the pit of my stomach. It had started to feel as if my insides had been twisted and wrapped around each other, the slightest thing that entered this twisted mess would have probably come back out spraying everywhere out of my mouth and nose. My hands were starting to feel a little clammy and I could feel beads of sweat starting to appear on my forehead. Taking a seat I was trying to keep myself calm, and normal. But today was far from normal.

Whilst exchanging small talk with Roger and Mary, Sandy went and pried Gordon away from his game playing. No doubt he was whooping someone's ass on Fifa. I could hear him upstairs asking for for a few more minutes, but his mother was telling him to come away and come downstairs. Of course he wouldn't be happy with that, once a game starts you can't just stop, that's absurd! Within a short space of time I could hear the clunking of his foot steps as he came downstairs. The stairs landed down into the dining area, this being an open plan front room and dining room type thing. As soon as he stepped out into the dining room he gazed across and saw us sitting on the sofa. He gave a slight, slightly confused smile.

"Dad what are you doing here? You're not supposed to be here until Friday and it's only Thursday?"

His voice was a mixture of being happy to see me, but he didn't understand why I was here.

"Is Granddad in hospital again? Is he okay?"

I guess that question said a lot about how many times my father had been in and out of hospital!

"Yes Granddad's okay, he's at home."

This conversation was a little bit awkward and I really didn't know in which direction to take it, but then there it came.

"Daddy needs to tell you something." Sandy's voice came across from the other side of the room.

"Oh okay, that's a bit strange. What do you want?" Gordon replied.

"Come over here and I'll tell you." I beckoned Gordon over to sit by my side. As he came across he gave me a quick hug and sat next to me.

"What's Grandma doing here as well?"

And so it began.

"Well Gordon, you know I wasn't very well that time when I was off work for along time, and you know I sometimes don't feel all that great?"

"Yes."

"Okay, well, I've been to see some nice people at the hospital today and they have told me something. They were trying to find out why I was poorly, they took some blood and they have found something."

My mind was quickly trying to work out a way to explain it simply without scaring him, and doing it in a way so that he would perhaps understand. Not an easy task but I had to think fast and think like a ten year old.

"What have they found?" Gordon's eyes were transfixed on me inquisitively.

"Well" I hesitated for a second, then suddenly it came

out. "They have found out that I'm not like everyone else ... I'm slightly different. You know the X-men right?"

"Yeah of course I do." Gordon replied a little confused.

"I have a mutation that makes me like an X-man."

"So you have superpowers?"

"Not quite, it's a little bit different to that. It would be nice to have superpowers, but it's because of that, that I'm not very well sometimes and can't always play football with you all the time."

"Oh ok. It would have been cool if you did have superpowers though wouldn't it."

"Yes, if I could shoot laser beams out of my eyes then that would have been excellent."

"I suppose if you're one of the X-men though that's still quite good .. what does it mean though Dad?"

"It basically just means I have to be a little more careful than everyone else. No different to now really, but the people at the hospital would also like to check your blood as well, to see if you are like me."

"So I could be one of the X-men too?"

"I don't think you are, but they just want to be sure, is that okay?"

"Yeah I guess so. Is Grandad one of the X-men too?"

"Yes, he is."

"Okay, well I don't mind being an X-man if you both are."

"Alright then, well when we get the appointment sorted we will take you, and they will have a look at your blood too."

"Yeah alright. Are you still coming to pick me up tomorrow for the weekend?"

"Of course, my boy!"

I'm not exactly sure how I suddenly came to describing myself being like one of the X-men, but if you think about it, it is right in a way, I'm a mutant. There is a mutation in my DNA that makes me different to everyone else. In essence that is the same as being one of the X-men, just without the superpowers and a bit of a crappy mutation! Looking back I think it turned out all right, explaining it so that he wouldn't be scared of having the blood test done, explaining it so he knew something was wrong but without having to go into all the details. When he is older I'm sure he will learn about the severity of what being one of the X-men means, but for now, that was all that was needed and would help him to understand.

So this day had perhaps been one of the longest and most memorable of my time here on this world. A great mystery had unfolded, the pieces of the puzzle had been put into place. Answers to questions had been found. But did these answers really serve any purpose? Nothing had really changed, except the fact that we now had a name for the evil inside. The enemy that we had always unknowingly battled. Vascular Ehlers-Danlos.

3

Now for everything bad that happens there is a good that happens. There has to be balance in the world to keep things even. In times of darkness, there is always a light lingering somewhere waiting to be switched on. For every act of cruelty, there is an act of kindness, there's good and evil in this world. I may have said this before and even now I still believe that everything happens for a reason. There are occurrences in life that are perhaps just meant to be. Against all the odds, things just happen. The next part of my story could perhaps be a whole story in itself. In fact we may just make it a story one day, for that you will have to wait and see. In this time of darkness, a light had began to flicker, which would turn into a full on shining star. What was about to take place was the forming of a bond that defies all odds. A chance meeting that would form a bond that will last until the end of time. For those of you that were paying attention, then you will have noticed that on this eventful day August the 22nd, you will remember that miles away another event was yet to take place and here it is!

That evening when the day was winding down, I couldn't sleep. I didn't really know what to think. None of it felt real, it still felt like a nightmare. The future had changed into something uncertain, a fear of the unknown. Darkness filling my life. I didn't know what would lie ahead. It's amazing how your life can be changed in a heartbeat. I sat around, thinking, but not really thinking. Sat looking through my window at the world outside wondering what the future would hold. Is there even going to be a future? What happens now? There is nothing to be done to fight this thing inside of me, there is nothing I can do to stop the inevitable. It will strike whenever and wherever it wants to and there is nothing, absolutely nothing that can be done. So what is my next move in this crazy game of life.

Eventually I got my sleep and the day ended. The next day I was back at work, carrying on as normal as if nothing had happened. Trying to work through it in my head but not knowing what to make of it. It seemed easier than I thought it would be. Just another normal day, as if the events of the day before had never happened. It was quite strange to have such a normal day when the previous had marked such a momentous occasion. It was a little awkward to concentrate I have to say. My mind I suppose was a little dazed and kept drifting back over and over different things. But then I would get busy and it would be forgotten about again. That was of course until I left work and was back in the confines of my own home and on my own. Then I had time to think and I decided to seek out others of my kind.

I found myself on the Ehlers-Danlos forum, and decided to post a message. It was a pretty simple message stating that I was newly diagnosed and was looking for other people in the same boat. The next day I got a reply, from someone that was to become the biggest light in my life. A bond was about to be formed that I could have never imagined.

Her name was Pink Lily. Surprisingly it turned out that she had also had a positive blood test for vEDS from Sheffield the same week as myself. Now the last time I heard, there were only around one hundred people in the UK diagnosed with vEDS. Out of all the people in this country of ours, around 64 million according to Google, the odds of finding someone diagnosed with vEDS the same week were pretty slim. The message board didn't even really have that many posts. According to statistics there are only ten people being diagnosed in the time span of a year in the UK. So many things had to have happened to bring us both to that place, to enable us to find that place, and find each other.

Do I believe in fate? Well I don't know, but as time has gone by and how close we have become from that very first day maybe it's more than just chance. Maybe this was mapped out generations before we were even born, millions and trillions of small events and decisions being made all leading down to the place we were meant to be. Perhaps this path has been written and we are all just playing the roles that are decided for us. What would have happened if my appointment had been a day later, or a day earlier, would I have still gone on that message board, would we have started talking to each other? Would we have met later on down the line? We will never know, but if there was a positive to be had from what was happening through all this mess. Then this was it. Pink Lily.

Straying from the time line to tell you a little more, I have now known Pink Lily for just over a year and four months. There has hardly been a day gone by that we haven't spoken to each other in some way. She lives many miles away from me, all the way down past London. It has come to be that I feel like she is family. Pink Lily has been there from the beginning of the diagnosis, sharing the ups and the downs. I would even say she now probably knows me better than anyone. We have laughed together, cried together. Mentally she has become my rock, and has helped to keep me moving forward when all I want to do is stop. In my darkest hours, Pink Lily has been my light and I know that we will continue to be friends for the rest of our lives. I still haven't met her yet, through work and life time seems to quickly slip through your fingers. But I aim to change this quite soon, when my work here is done, I shall be going to meet her, her husband and her daughter, with a copy of this book in hand, because in the background she has also been spurring me on to continue writing this!

So what does Pink Lily look like you ask? Well, she is beautiful, long straight blond hair, big smiley eyes, with the most amazing sense of humour, although how many times she is going to take the piss out of my pronunciation of "duck", I do not know. Apparently, my Lincolnshire accent, not that I think I have one, makes it sound like "dook". But then I do tend to think her pronunciation sounds a little like "dack", so I have a little ammo to fight back with!

Together we have started on a path to gain knowledge,

seeking out others in the same situation. We have helped each other get the tools we need to try and keep us and our families as safe as we possibly can. There is no cure, but at least we can know what to look for, and know the people to speak to. When you are diagnosed with something like this, its good that you have friends around you, but they can never really understand. To connect with somebody who is in the same position and going through the same emotions is the work of miracles!

There are so many tales I would like to tell you about the ways in which our friendship has grown. But I fear if I started to go into a full run down, then I would be far diverted away from the tale at hand. In truth, I really don't know how to convey how important a role Pink Lily and her family have come to play! I could never ever do it justice with my amateur skills, although as the story unfolds perhaps you will see how this has come to be! There is one small tale that I would like to share with you though and here it is!

Meerkats, a little like Marmite. You either love them or you hate them. Well it just happens that for some strange reason, I love them.

"Have you ever seen me dancing? You know .. REALLY dancing?"

How can one not like that classic line that rolls off the meerkat's tongue in the famous television advert for "Clorets" I think it was, if my memory serves me right.

I think this was the advert that made meerkats become the animal equivalent to Marmite. In my mind it was anyway.

Anyhow, I had a toy meerkat, a stuffed fluffy one at that, which I had named Meredith. This may sound a little bit wacky or downright bizarre to some people, but for me, it was the normal sort of thing that I did. I packed up Meredith in a box, very carefully and sent her on her 2013 Christmas holidays down to Pink Lily's. I thought if nothing else then it would give Pink Lily and her family a little to smile and laugh about.

What happened next was one of the most amazing things that possibly could happen to a fluffy toy. Meredith had been with Pink Lily for a few days, I was constantly being sent pictures of her adventures, which seemed fantastic. Meredith was fitting right in at home with the Pink Lily family, she was even playing games of hide and seek in the Christmas tree.

One day I received a very unexpected picture, Meredith had met another meerkat of the male variety. This did did worry me a little as Meredith was still young, although after speaking to Pink Lily it was clear that this male meerkat only had good intentions and was of very good character. Together they set off on a fluffy meerkat romance and in the weeks to follow I received some more news. Meredith was pregnant, but more than that, she had already had the babies. It was a little shocking at first, but from the pictures that Pink Lily sent I could see they were very happy together. Meredith had even gone out to get a job to support her family.

At this point it was clear that Meredith wouldn't be coming back home again, but that was okay, she had found love, started a family and was being responsible about the whole situation. Not only that, Meredith was in the greatest of hands, a better home than I could have ever offered her. One day hopefully I will see her again and meet her children, but until that day I know she is safe just where she is.

4

So here we are, on day two after being fully fledged diagnosed. The sun had set the night before and the sun arose once again in the morning. The world around me hadn't changed, I hadn't changed, but everything HAD changed. But what did I feel? I felt nothing, I felt everything. I was numb, I was scared. I was angry, I was frustrated, yet my mind was empty. Confusion, a blank expression, dazed. It was one big mess of nothingness. Can this emotion really be explained? I'm not so sure it can unless you feel it for yourself.

For now we just had to carry on. The start of this journey had begun many many years before, passed down from generation to generation, how far back it goes we will probably never know, but this was where it had led us today. Again it makes me think that maybe this is all a predetermined plot we are playing out. Going about our lives, making choices that take us to the places we are supposed to be. But really, who would want to find themselves on this path? There were more hard times to come, this was for certain.

The next step was for Gordon to be tested. I went once again to work as usual that day, just another normal day of wandering around aimlessly amidst the madness. Now the doctor hadn't called back last night, it was late I guess so this was to be expected. But within a few hours of being at work I had a phone call.

"Hello."

"Hi Dave, its Sandy. The doctor rang and asked for us to go in, and we have an appointment in a few hours."

"Okay well let me know how you get on."

The phone went down. Short and sweet. It had to be really, there was nothing left to say. The gravity of the situation was growing on the shoulders. I had been so dazed and empty this morning but with that phone call, there was something brewing up that I didn't like. I was starting to realise that my child was in danger. Real danger. And this was something I wouldn't be able to protect him from. If I felt this, she must have felt it too.

His mother Sandy must be feeling that uncertainty. I think a part of me could hear it in her voice, but maybe not, either way I didn't want the doubt in my mind to be known, somehow I had to hide it.

As the time ticked by slowly, again the phone rang.

"Hi, its Sandy again." Her voice seemed surprisingly normal.

"How's it going?" I eagerly wanted to hear.

"The doctor didn't know what vEDS was."

"No surprise there then!"

"But he did Google it, and said how serious it was."

"Okay, so ..?"

"He wrote the referral off while I was there and he's going to post it personally so he knows it's gone and will get there quick."

"That's excellent, hopefully it won't be too long."

It felt a little more refreshing that someone was understanding the urgency.

"What time will you be picking up Gordon tonight?"

"Will be the usual time as soon as I get out of here."

"Okay, I'll have him ready."

With that it was over. I was quite relieved it was a little easier getting Gordon across there. This didn't need to be strung out any longer than it should. Waiting for the blood test back for him was going to be long enough itself. Not a challenge that I really wanted to go through.

As normal I picked Gordon up that night. The weekend was like any other really. Gordon didn't make much of what I had told him the previous night. There were a few questions, but nothing too serious and he seemed to be okay with everything. There would be questions further down the line, this I was certain of, but now they could stay on the back burner as I didn't want him to have to carry this burden. I remember when I was younger, I was a few years older than Gordon mind, my father had his first heart attack, the first of many domino effects. A day that would eventually lead to a world of seeing the inside of too many hospitals.

There was one thing that did change that weekend. I looked at Gordon more. Without even realising it I was looking at everything, every movement, and I began to see things. I began to see things that I didn't like. Those little pointers. How many bruises has he got? Does he look to bruise easily? No, impossible, it's impossible to tell right? He's ten, all ten year-olds have bruises. Doubt was entering my mind, creeping up to fill the emptiness that I was feeling. A fear, an almost instant panic. Mentally making a check box in my head, then telling myself "No way". It can't be, it won't be. I had to keep control of it, keep it in check. This wouldn't last long, it would soon be over. He'll be okay and then everything else will be okay.

It didn't take long for the letter to come through. Within a week we had an appointment. I was grateful that they were moving it along so quickly, when your child's life is threatened with something so horrible. A curse so harsh and unpredictable that was plaguing us all, to think that I could have passed this on to him was starting to eat at me. I would look back on my life and deep down I always knew. I always knew there was something there. All the scans they gave me for the HCM would come back negative but still I would believe something was there. I could feel it sometimes, even though I didn't really know, I did know. That gut feeling. My gut feelings are rarely wrong!

5

The day had come round. It was time to take Gordon once again to the place I had grown not to like. To get in my trusty Focus and travel the road towards the place of answers. By now I was sure that my car was beginning to learn to drive this road itself.

It was a morning appointment, so no lengthy waiting around. Straight there and straight in, of course the answers still wouldn't be quite there but perhaps we would have a better idea of how this was going to pan out. I was hoping that once they had seen Gordon that it would be ruled out clinically straight away. This would have been a great weight lifted off the shoulders. Two weeks had begun to take their toll. Sleepless nights had been many. I still didn't feel anything about myself, the only concerns I had were now shifted and focused on Gordon. Time and time again I had spoken to my parents who would reassure me that they didn't think he looked like he had it, I even tried to convince myself, although I could still see those signs, niggling away at me time and time again. Denying them access and trying to stay positive.

As we arrived at the hospital nothing much had changed. It had been but a few weeks that I had been there. Everything was still the same, the same old old buzzer system to get in the door, the same warm welcome that I had earlier received. Only this time, I didn't really feel it. I could feel an urgency inside of me, I just wanted this to be over.

As we sat down down in the reception I felt cold. The place was empty and it was pretty silent. I could hear the clock ticking above my head, every second seeming to last a minute. I'd obviously learnt from the day the camera was shoved down my throat that there were in actual fact sixty seconds in a minute. But now there seemed to be more. It was starting to feel as though time had been expanded. The days were the same, and yet they had grown longer. It was like sitting in front of a VCR, pressing the pause button and then watching the world go by one frame at a time. This was something I did on a regular occasion on the old VCR. It's amazing the simple amusements that the mind creates. I remember watching a scene out of "Cobra", for those of you that don't remember, it was a Sylvester Stallone classic that takes a place in my ever expanding DVD collection. In it there was a scene where Stallone was riding a motorbike down the road, I would pause and rewind it to watch him ride backwards. It is definitely a feature that is lacking in DVD players.

After what seemed like hours, finally I heard footsteps coming from down the corridor. To me they sounded like footsteps with purpose. They were nicely evenly paced, well, that was until suddenly there seemed to be some sort of stumble. As I heard this I looked at Gordon and my face broke into a little smile. He let out a hidden chuckle, perhaps as though he had imagined the poor soul had taken on a bit of wobble. I cannot begin to imagine what was actually running through his mind. If he was scared then he hid it very well indeed.

"Good morning David, it's nice to see you again." came the voice of Rosemary as she appeared from out of the corridor where we had heard the footsteps. Little did she know Gordon and I were very well aware of her little mis-step.

"Good morning, how are you?"

"Oh you know, just another manic Monday." Rosemary's reply reminded me of a song but I refrained.

"And I take it this is Gordon? He looks like you." Her eyes this time had been transfixed on Gordon as she had come round, which I noticed very closely. I had a feeling I would be taking in every little detail this time. Alertness of what may be coming was my aim.

The fact that Rosemary had stated Gordon looked like me was not to my liking, I didn't want him to look like me and nor did I want him to be anything to be like me. Not at this point. I still truly didn't understand what all of this meant, but even so. I really didn't want this for him.

"Yes, this is my boy."

"Hello." was his shy, short reply, slightly hiding whilst sat between his mother and I.

"And this must be Gordon's mother, Sandy isn't it?" Her voice was soft and almost sympathetic.

"Hi, yes I'm Sandy, nice to meet you."

"Okay well, would you like to come through?"

With that, Rosemary motioned her arms towards the corridor on the right. Leading the way, we were once again taken into the room that I had now been in twice. The same window looked at me, the one with the greatest of views, the bricks, oh so many bricks that I had drifted off and counted before. In reality it was a bit of a poor excuse for a window. There was a distinct lack of light that it let in. Somehow it was beginning to feel like a jail cell.

As I walked in, Gordon behind me, then Sandy and Rosemary leading the way, I was suddenly hit by a memory. The memory of Rosemary reaching across and touching my leg, the eyes upon me waiting to see if I would breakdown and cry with the words they had just uttered.

"You have a mutation."

No, no, no, no! That goes in the little lock box. It stays there firmly shut for the minute. We will contend with that later. Now is the time to keep my cool and not let anything affect me. My mind is strong, my mind is focused, there are more important issues at hand.

Sitting in that same chair, with the same layout, there was Dr Gazelle Banger. She was writing up some notes. As we walked through the door, Rosemary closing it behind us, Gazelle slowly looked up and without saying a word beckoned us to take our seats. This we followed and Dr Banger slowly brought her attention to the three people before her.

"Good morning David. Thankyou for coming again and bringing Gordon."

And there it was, that soft voice, but a faint whisper travelling through the air.

"So Gordon," Her eyes, as with Rosemary's were transfixed on Gordon, "Do you know why you are here? What has your father told you?"

Woah, was this some sort of test to see what my fatherhood abilities were like. Please don't tell me they want him to know the full story.

"Hi."

Gordon let out a little smile, adjusting himself in his seat slightly, legs dangling awkwardly from the chair.

"Well .." followed by a slight pause while he turned to look at me.

"It's okay, you can speak to them." I looked at him and smiled.

"Well .. you want to have a look at me .. and take some blood to test?" His answer was correct but he was still a little unsure.

"Yes that's right" replied Gazelle. "Your dad has a mutation in his genes that we want to rule out in you, its that okay?"

Gordon was silent for a minute, looking around the room, but never at the pair of eyes that were set upon him. He turned to his mother, then back towards to me, back down to his feet, and then raised his head slightly and began to talk.

"That's okay, will it hurt taking the blood out?" He spoke quietly. Whilst he had had blood tests before, he knew this one was a little different.

Rosemary smiled at Gordon and in a quiet reassuring voice said, "It won't hurt, you'll feel a tiny pinch that's all, and I'm sure Mummy or Daddy will keep you occupied so you don't notice it." Her head raised slightly and looked at Sandy and I.

With that, Rosemary slowly got up from her chair.

"Gordon, would you like to come through and put a night gown on so we can take a look at you. Mum or Dad can come through with you."

"OK, Dad you can come."

And with that I also rose to my feet and took Gordon through to the back room.

Rosemary reached for a nicely fashioned chequered hospital gown and left the room so that Gordon could get undressed. Slowly he took off his clothes and said,

"Do I really have to wear this dad, I'm going to look an idiot" as he chuckled.

"That's the latest hospital fashion my child! You will be fine." I replied, slightly laughing.

As he slipped it on there came a knock at the door.

"Are we all fit?" came Rosemary's voice,

"Yep, all ready," replied Gordon.

The door opened and in came Rosemary, followed by Dr Banger who was armed with her clipboard and pen. I could see the check-sheet attached to the board. I knew exactly how this went.

I stepped to the side and let Dr Banger move towards Gordon. Slowly she began going through the inspection, item by item. Holding out his arms, bending the tips of his fingers back, turning over the hands, moving up to the elbow, pulling at the skin. The same routine that she had done on myself previously. I watched her attentively, every time she moved her eyes I would follow straight to were she was looking, every time she marked something down I would make a mental note in my head. Slowly summing everything up. As her eyes moved from his chest to the back of his shoulders, noting the visible veins under his skin. The more I watched her the more I began to see the signs. I found myself piecing it all together once again, just like I had back when I took my checklist to the doctor.

Dr Banger stepped back from Gordon. It was time to test his gymnastic ability.

"Okay Gordon, could you stretch down and place your hands on the floor without bending your knees?"

With that Gordon bent down and placed his hands on the floor in a squat.

"Like that?"

"No, Gordon, not quite like that, don't bend your knees." I told him with a smile on my face.

"I don't know what you mean?"

"I'd best show you then." I said as I stepped forward, legs straightened and started to bend forward with arms outreached towards the floor.

"But you can't do it Dad."

"I know, it's okay. You don't have to be able to do it, just give it a try and see if you can."

Gordon then locked his knees in place, and slowly he bent his back and pushed his arms forward toward the floor. I could tell he really wanted to outdo me and place his hands on the cold floor. He tried two or three times, but nope, he couldn't do it! As he rose back up he started to shake his head with disappointment in the fact that he couldn't do it.

Rosemary let out a chuckle, "Its okay Gordon, it wasn't a competition. We are all done now, we just want to take a few pictures now if that's okay, for our records?"

"Yeah alright," he replied.

Dr Banger then left the room along with her check sheet and left Rosemary to take a few snaps. When she was done Gordon got dressed again and we went out back into the office area.

Sandy was sitting there, still with a slight look of concern in her eyes. Dr Banger hadn't spoken to her while she finished up writing her notes. We all sat down again, in silence for a few moments. I watched Dr

Banger as she scribbled around with her pen, seeing the lines of ink coming out of the pen as I followed it sharply with my eyes. For a moment it was as if I could see the pen moving around in slow motion, smoothly gliding across the paper. Then after a few more silent minutes Dr Banger looked right back at us.

"Well, as you know David, like we did with you we can usually give a good indication on the basis of the visual exam, although in Gordon's case I'm afraid we can't do that. He does tick a lot of the boxes. There are some visible veins, he has over extendibility in his finger tips and also in his elbows slightly. Unfortunately it is inconclusive and we will have to take the blood sample, send that away and rule it out like that. It won't however take as long as to come back as we know what to look for rather than having to check the whole DNA sequence."

"Okay so how long do you think it will be and what do you think the chances are if you were to take a guess?"

"Well we really can't guess. We will have to wait for the bloodwork to come back. I will put a special note on and make sure it gets looked at straight away. We should know within three to four weeks, all being well."

"Well, we'd best get some blood then hadn't we? You okay with that Gordon?" I shifted my gaze towards my son, he looked remarkably calm.

"That's okay. As long as it's not going to hurt."

"No don't worry Gordon, I will be gentle with you!" Rosemary said in a reassuring voice.

Going back into the examination room Gordon jumped onto the bed. He sat there with his sleeves rolled up and his arms outstretched, ready and waiting, but not looking anywhere near the needle. Rosemary was true to her word and very gentle. No messing around, in went the needle, out came the blood. She made it seem so simple, which impressed me quite a bit. I was always used to people digging around trying to find an entrance into myself. Pricking me and tapping me to try and make the veins arise from underneath.

On the ride home, Gordon was pretty quiet, in fact we all were. I was very much hoping that we would have gotten a "no" there and then. An answer either way would have been better. Now though, it was back to the waiting game. Everything always seems to be a waiting game. They say that patience is a virtue, well after all the recent events and the time that was passing by, my patience was wearing a little thin. When you're waiting for something like this, the world carries on around you, but the time goes by oh so slowly! You feel every torturous second, your mind doubting, then trying to rid yourself of the doubt. It's a non stop merry go round. Backwards and forwards in your head constantly. You try to sleep, but as soon as you lie down the mind becomes an explosion of thoughts. Relentless until you finally drift away into the dark abyss. Sometimes I wish I could go back to the times when everything was simple. But no, the journey had to be played out.

6

Time. Time is a bizarre concept. He who controls time controls the world? Maybe, maybe not. Perhaps you are getting a little bored about me rambling on about time, but bear with me. Hey, I now have another three to four weeks to wait. So lets have a little ponder while I sit here and run my hands through my silky soft beard .. The origin of time itself was the Big Bang, perhaps. Did time exist before this? Maybe it did but we didn't have the ability to measure it. Twenty-four hours in a day came from the ancient Egyptians. The sixty seconds in an hour was from the ancient Babylonians.

Well, so that's what Google says. But is time really equal. Do we not measure time ourselves based on the way we feel. They say when you're having fun time flies, which it does. But why? Why is that one hour can pass by so fast, when another hour can pass by so slowly. There is no difference in the measurement. One hour remains one hour no matter what. It's a constant that has been around for years, yet the feeling of time seems to alter depending on our feelings, our moods and our activities. So in actual fact does this not mean that we ourselves are the masters of time. Maybe we are all just timelords, Dr Who's in our own rights, our minds and feelings like a Tardis.

What about another timeline that runs parallel to the constant of conventional time. Forget the whole twenty-four hours in a day, and sixty minutes in an hour. What if there was a timeline that we control. You look at people at the age of say sixty, some don't look a day over what normal time would call fifty, yet others look like what we could call seventy. So is there another time line that lies within us? For those that look younger than they are, have they managed to find a way to slow down the ageing process. Our minds have powers that perhaps we don't even know we have and could never realise. Perhaps I'm just babbling. But maybe, just maybe I'm onto something.

So really, what is this about you might ask? Well okay all this waiting around. Waiting for results to come back time and time again. These aren't the hours that fly by when you are having fun. These are the hours that drag on and on and on, sixty minutes in an hour doesn't seem like an accurate measurement. Three or four weeks was feeling more like three or four months. When time is a constant, how is that possible? These are life defining moments. The world isn't changing, but your world is. Your life and that of those you love, is changing. Sure, there are many bad things in this world and many people in worse places. But this, this is your life. No one else's; its yours, your situation. You are trapped in it and there is no escape. And that damn time ticks by so slowly, whilst in the world around you everything just carries on.

What now then? With these long ass minutes, what was I supposed to do? The usual. I would go to work, keep busy and everything was normal. Just carrying on as if nothing was happening. The days would end and I'd jump in to my bed and bang! I'm not sleeping, I'm turning over backwards and forwards waiting. The days were not too bad. But the nights! It was the nights that would drag on even further. I tried a little to ignore it, but I couldn't. It was during these nights that I began to look again. So Google would play a big role in the next few weeks and so did Pink Lily. We were in contact most of the time, sometimes talking seriously, but then sometimes talking about complete and utter rubbish, not rubbish, but you know what I mean. The endless conversations that you have between friends that just seem crazy. Just totally random things.

How did I do with Google and searching? It was exhausting. How many times can you type in Vascular Ehlers-Danlos Syndrome and come up with nothing. Because there really was nothing. Case studies here and there, but meaningless. There were no answers for anything, just endless amounts of questions. Backwards and forwards, I would go over it time and time again. I was beginning to feel powerless. There was nothing I could do, nothing. Until one night when I was lying in the bath browsing on my phone. I came across an article relating to a lady in America. Research. Interesting. This lady went by the name of Gwen Patroni. The article that

I read stated that she was very well versed in Ehlers-Danlos, but more so in Vascular Ehlers-Danlos. Perhaps this was what I was looking for. Would I find my answers here? I hoped so. Gwen was beginning research into Vascular Ehlers-Danlos and collecting samples. I can't remember the ins and outs of what I found now, as you know, my memory isn't that great. But it didn't matter. I found something. I was too tired to do anything more, remember, these days were long as I was still waiting for the results. So with that in mind I left it there for the evening.

The very next day I went to work as usual, feeling just a tad better about myself for possibly stumbling on to something. I think my work colleagues may have noticed. I hadn't really been myself for a while, but at least today there was a hint of myself coming through. A little later in the day, another most bizarre thing happened, a very strange coincidence. Pink Lily sent me through a very excited text. She told of how she had just finished Skypeing, can you guess? Well if you can't, it just so happened to be the American lady Gwen Patroni. Pink Lily mentioned how she was doing research and was well versed in vEDS. I was amazed, there I was in the bath finding this person and at the same time Pink Lily had also found the same thing and got into contact with her. Fantastic!

Pink Lily had spoken to Gwen about my current situation and was advised to give me Gwen's contact details. Across the ocean there was someone out there looking out for us. Not only that, there was some sort of research going on that I could be part of. Perhaps this could be a route to finding a way to fight against this. In this moment I felt a great sense of hope.

That night as soon as I arrived home I switched on the PC, and sent an email to Gwen. In this email I included my specific mutation.

p.[9Gly252Val0];[=]

This was what was written in the findings of the blood test. It meant nothing at all to me. Why on earth would it? I had learnt a little about genetics and biology back in the school days, but back then none of this really interested me and how could I have known that one day it could have helped me. I was more into my english, and business studies. Apparently this was the mutation of the collagen that was found within. A whole set of random numbers and letters. I mentioned a brief description of what had come to pass, the tale of how it had been in our family for years, but had never been mentioned until I had my problems. I mentioned how I was waiting for my son's test to come back and how I wanted to help in some way, shape or form in finding something to control this. I mentioned that I had heard about the research she had been doing, and wanted to be part of this, and that I wanted to keep hope alive.

Obviously with our time differences I didn't receive a reply straight away. I wasn't all that sure I would get a reply for days, weeks maybe. In Gwen's position I could only imagine that she was very busy. She probably had hundreds of people all over the world emailing her just like me. All seeking out help in their time of darkness. All looking for that little ray of light to keep hope afloat. We shall talk about that word hope a little later!

Okay so, the email was sent. Now, again, all I had to do was wait. I can happily tell you that the wait wasn't long. In fact, the very next day I received an email back from Gwen. It was short, but amazing. When you're walking through the unknown and someone reaches out their hand to help you, you take it.

"Hi David, thank-you for your email. Do you have

Skype, can you add me so that we can talk. My user id is Gwen Patroni."

The email came in the morning while I was working. With this new found excitement distracting me from what was happening I couldn't wait. I made arrangements to have the afternoon off so that I could pursue this further. Suddenly there had become an urgency inside of me. I needed answers, I needed something. Everything was hanging in the balance.

When I arrived home I shot straight up the stairs, tripping upwards as I defied the laws of gravity once again. I seemed to have a knack of not quite lifting my leg up far enough to clear the last step I was going up. My foot would slightly catch the step and I would be tossed forward letting out an immediate cry:

"Woah, shit!"

How many times I have done this I cannot tell you. But I can tell you that I always came down with a thud, throwing my arms out in front of me to stop my face planting into the hardness of the stairs. If I was ever to go down, it would leave me in a bloody mess. Instead it is usually my wrist that gets the full brunt of the force. Smacking down hard on the corner of the stair, resulting in a burst vein time and time again. For the days to follow the bruise would eventually form out to leave my wrists black, looking as though I had been kidnapped and tied up by the evilness that is the Kung Fu squirrels!

I chuckled as I got up and brushed myself off and headed straight towards the PC. Pressing the power on, it was seconds before it booted up and was ready to use. Ten seconds to be precise. Remember I enjoyed building computers, well mine is a powerhouse, complete with one of the fastest solid state drives you could have. Before SSDs, you could put the kettle on and almost make a full cup of tea. With the advancement of technology though, you didn't even have time to boil the water!

Loading up Skype I entered the contact ID for Gwen. My request of an add was soon accepted, and there was Gwen's name highlighted in green to show an online presence. Seeing this I quickly typed a chat message:

"Hi it's David, thankyou for wanting to speak to me, is now a good time?"

"Yep, now is an excellent time, just give me ten minutes."

Jumping out of my seat I went across the room to flick the kettle. I don't think I had ever been so eager to Skype with someone. I'm not really a lover of video messaging or phone calls. I prefer to be stood in front of someone talking to them. A phone call only gives half a conversation, or perhaps even less. I like to be able to see the body language that goes along with the words. The only reason I had Skype was to stay in contact with my brother in Germany, it was free, it was easy.

As I returned to my seat, cup of tea in hand, the distinctive ring of an inbound Skype call was coming through my speakers, I hovered the cursor over to the answer with video button and clicked. For a few seconds there was complete black, and then the screen came to life.

There in front me was a room. Not one of an office that I was expecting to see, but that of a dining room. A table in the middle with books and papers piled up over it. A cat sat on top staring back and me. Bookcases in the background filled with what looked like a mixture of medical research books and endless novels.

A voice came from nowhere in the background.

"Hi David, I'll be with you in one minute."

As a figure came around from the side of the camera, the first thing I noticed was the smile. It was warm and most welcoming, not a fake smile, because she had the eyes to match. Gwen really did seem to be pleased to be talking to me. I also noticed her hair, really bushy black hair, slightly wavy, flowing down to her neck. As she got comfy in her seat she began to speak.

"Hi David, sorry about that, I was just feeding the cat to distract it. Its really nice to meet you. Lily has told me a lot about you, how are you doing."

"I'm not bad all things considered. Still a little bit numb at the minute I guess."

"Well it's not a small thing that's happening. I'm quite relieved that you got in contact, from your email it sounds like you have been going through it a little bit. Hows your father?"

"He's not too bad at the minute, in fact he's doing quite well."

"Okay that's good, and what about your son, how's he handling this?"

"As far as I can tell, he seems to be all right. I haven't told him that much about what's going on. I just told him that I was an X-man of sorts and we just needed to test him. He knows I haven't been too well and with the problems that my father's had he is sort of used to it, well as much as you can be I suppose."

"One of the X-men, that's one way of putting it. Good thinking! It does take a little time to make sense of it all though. I was quite impressed that you found out about vEDS after all those years of your father having problems. Unfortunately that is often the case with something like this. It is easily missed. The figures you have probably read are nowhere near what they should be because there isn't enough awareness out there. We are making some headway though, and having a diagnosis really can make a difference. There is some great research going on and we hope to make advances very soon. I see hundreds of patients with Ehlers-Danlos Syndrome as well as Marfans Syndrome, and I even see a lot of people with Vascular type. The problem is, most doctors will have heard about Ehlers-Danlos in general, but it would be very rare for a doctor to see anyone diagnosed with Vascular type in their lifetime."

Gwens tone was excitable and happy, you could really tell that her heart was in this. This wasn't just a job to her, but a way of life. I think she is one of those people that just wants to help people, and she was in the position to do it.

"Yes it does seem to be very rare and nobody seems to know anything about it. I've been looking on the internet but everything I seem to find leads to badness."

"The main reason for that is because often the diagnosis isn't made until after something major has happened. The life expectancy for instance is based on figures from people that have been diagnosed. There are more people out there that will have gone through their lives without being diagnosed and lived to a ripe old age."

"Yes, my father is sixty soon. It's a been a long slog, but he keeps going strong and defying the odds."

"He sounds like an amazing man. So is there anything you would like to ask me?"

"The research. I heard that you are signing up people to take part in it and I would like to be a part of it. I know myself that it's not going to help me, but if it can help future generations then I am more than willing to do whatever it takes."

"Of course you can. The more people we sign up and the more information about vEDS we can collate, the better. You're just in time as well as I only have two more weeks to get people to sign up. I should be able to get a kit out for you straight away. What I will need you to do is send the kit back to me as soon as you get it. It's just a swab kit so that we can take a sample of your DNA to study the mutation. From what you sent the mutation you have is quite a common one. I will send you some forms to fill out. If you can take a look and sign them, then get them back to me that would be great. They are just forms so that we can send to your doctors to ask them to release any previous scan results."

"That would be excellent, I will do that as soon as I receive them, it feels good to be able to do something."

I was very impressed, this was putting a positive into the negative. I didn't quite feel so helpless about the situation now.

"If you email me your full address then I will get that done right away for you."

"Thanks, I'll send my address across as soon as we finish on here."

"Now with regard to vEDS itself, is there anything you would like to you know?"

Gwen leaned forward and waited for my answer, eyes wide open and ready for anything.

"Well I've read a little bit as you know, but what can I do now I'm diagnosed, there doesn't seem to be any set in stone guidelines as to what I should or shouldn't do?" I asked.

"No, I'm afraid there aren't any real guidelines. But there are things that you can avoid to keep yourself safe and arming yourself with knowledge will help. In the case of vEDS, knowledge is power. It is unpredictable but if you know what to look out for it can help greatly. What tablets are you taking?"

With that I jumped up out of my seat and headed across to the pantry style cupboard, came back and reeled off the list of tablets.

"That's good. I do have a couple of suggestions though. Have you got your appointment through to see the cardiologist?"

"Yes I'm back there in a few weeks to see the cardiologist and EDS team again."

"Right, that's excellent. You're on the right path. It is very important to have a medical team together in the event of complications. If surgery is ever needed for whatever reason, then the doctors can talk to your medical team and be advised on procedures. Because the arteries are weaker and tear easily, operating can be a problem and should only be done in extreme situations, and you must have a vascular surgeon present no matter what."

Gwen continued. "Now, as for the tablets, I suggest you speak to them about the blood thinner. I understand that you have had a stroke, and they do help to avoid stroke. The only danger is that if a rupture occurs in the arteries then these can make the bleed worse, which is something that we don't want. Have you heard of Celiprolol David?"

"I have heard a little about it, something to do with a French study?"

"Yes, there have been trials of Celiprolol in vEDS. While the results haven't been conclusive we believe that it can have an effect in the slow down of arterial events. Most patients I have seen with vEDS I have advised to go onto this. The results are very promising. Talk to your vascular team about this as well. It is also very important to monitor your blood pressure. The lower the blood pressure then the less stress it puts on your arteries. In vEDS, a nice pressure to try and aim for is 110/70."

This woman was turning out to be a world of information.

"As for day to day tasks, you need to make sure you put as little strain on the vascular system as possible. That means no heavy lifting, and nothing that exerts you too much. You still need exercise though, so walking, swimming and bike riding are advisable. Of course you also need to make sure you avoid impact events. If you take part in any sports they need to be low impact, and no roller coasting riding, sudden sharp movements can lead to tears. Are you working at the minute?"

"Yeah I'm back at work now. I had a few months off when I had my dissection, but went back when things started dying down a little. I still obviously have the day to day issues, but they are manageable."

"Okay what do you work as?"

"I work in sales and fit the odd car tyres here and there."

"You FIT tyres?" Gwen's eyes widened and her neck strained forward in a moment of shock.

"Yes I do," I replied sheepishly.

"Are you CRAZY? After a dissection of the carotid artery and you're fitting tyres?"

"Yes I know, but it's all I've known for years and I do seem to enjoy it."

"Oh, no no no, you really shouldn't be doing that. Lifting anything heavy and instantaneous exertion is something that should definitely not be done. You cannot strain the vascular system, that is very important. Is there anything else you can do. You must seriously think about stopping this."

"Well, I don't really know. It has been in the back of my mind that I shouldn't be doing it, however I don't know what else I could do. I'm not one to sit in the office all day. I have been doing this for around fourteen years now."

"Please think about it. If you do anything, this could be the best thing to keep you safe. You must take it easy and stay safe, I cannot emphasise enough how important this is. I don't mean to frighten you but it is that important. Just please be careful and reconsider."

Her face was now one of concern and the smile had faded a little, it obviously worried her. The truth is I had thought about it a little. I mean after all it does make sense. Putting too much of a strain on something that is flawed is not a good idea and could have deadly consequences.

"I will think about it. At the minute though my main concern is about Gordon. I'm not too bothered about myself, I just want to know that he's going to be okay and that I can protect him."

Gwen's smile once again returned.

"I can tell you care about him. Hopefully he will be all right, but don't forget you have to look after yourself for his sake as well as your own. Now have you got a medical alert? It is always handy to wear some form of medical alert. That way if something was to happen then they would know about the vEDS. In cases of emergency, previous patient history is often not known, and if no-one is around to tell them about the vEDS then this could cause problems."

"I haven't got one yet, but the geneticists have given me the information booklet about getting one. I also carry around a medical emergency paper memo in my wallet."

"That's good to hear. Well you seem to be pretty sensible and have a little knowledge of what you are faced with. Everything seems to be going in the right direction and you're on the right path. I have to shoot off to work now, but if you send me your address I will send out the swab kit. Thank you again for getting in contact with me, it's really nice to hear from you."

"No thank you for talking to me. You don't know what it means to be able to talk to someone like you. The fact that there is someone out there working to help us is amazing. You are a god send and you seem to know more than anyone I have ever spoken to. Thank you for your time, I really appreciate it."

"That's okay, if you need anything else then just message me. I might take a while to get back to you but I will try and help you where I can. Goodbye David."

"Goodbye, and thank you Gwen."

The screen went blank. Wow. Where exactly had this lady come from? Who was this person? She was amazing, knowledgeable and passionate. This was amazing, not only had I just been speaking to one of the greatest vEDS minds in the world but she was also going to allow me to be part of something big. Perhaps this way I could do something better with my life. More than just working, but actually helping generations to come. I felt a little inspired and more hopeful. Knowing that people do care makes all the more difference. Today was a fantastic day and really lifted my spirits to a height that they hadn't been to in a long while. Of course I had to share this with Pink Lily, after all she had put me in contact with Gwen and I'm sure the same feelings were running through her mind.

7

As we carry on a few weeks into the story, I had sent my home address across to Gwen. The DNA swab kit still hadn't arrived, but I had expected it to take a while coming all the way from across the other side of the world. I'd been feeling a little better about the situation. It still didn't seem real though. My health wasn't too bad apart from the usual aches and pains, the odd episode of vision loss here and there but overall this thing inside of me didn't feel as it if existed. I felt like a normal everyday person.

During the course of the next few weeks my father had received a phone call from the EDS clinic. The results were not a big surprise. It was well expected and the clinical diagnosis had already been made. Positive. It was now official after all these years that he had

Vascular Ehlers-Danlos. It really made no difference to him, after all, it had been creating problem after problem after problem for years. So many heart attacks and dissections you could never list them all. So many times of being told he was not going to live and yet proving them all wrong.

What I have neglected to perhaps tell you is of my brother over in Germany. While all this was going on, he was over there hearing snippets of the events that were unfolding. He had been to see a doctor regarding getting tested himself. In my mind, I was certain that he didn't have it. Out of us three children he always seems to have been the physically stronger one. He didn't bruise like us that I knew of, and didn't seem to have the constraints of having a faulty foundations. Where I saw it as plain as day in my sister Franny, I didn't see it him him. I think I already knew beforehand that he would be okay. The EDS clinic had sent a copy of my results over to his doctor in Germany so that they could test him and search for the same mutation that I had. The results for him came back in no time. Negative. This was good news. It meant that he could get on with his life and start a family, something he wanted to do and with a negative result it meant that he could do this without having to worry about the possibility of passing on the curse.

So what of Gordon? Was his fate to be that of ours? Was he destined to have this thrust upon him? The geneticists had been uncertain, I was uncertain. Although I really hoped that this would not be true for him and clung onto that thought like my life depended on it. I didn't want to think that I would one day have to stop him doing the things he loves most. I didn't want to tell his teachers about this. For Gordon I wanted a normal life, the best life he could have without having to worry about the fact that in seconds it could be ripped apart. In a way I might have been lucky that the doctors hadn't found it in my father when I was younger. It allowed me to grow up as any normal kid would. Playing rough, messing about and joining in with everyone else. Perhaps it might have helped to stop the dissection, but would I have dared do half the things I had done when I was a child. If the result was positive I knew that his childhood would be stripped away. To keep him safe, to keep him alive, but at what cost? To live a life in fear and to not do the things that you really want to do. How far do you go to stay safe when you are but a child? What do you have to take away in an effort to save a life, yet live a life?

I remember back in my school days, playing a game called "British Bulldogs". Two ends of the playground. In the middle you would have one person who would have to tag you as you tried to get from one end to the other. We all used to play it and it was usually pretty rough.

You would start out at one end of the playground, our playground was concrete. A group of people stood there, getting ready to run as fast as they could, and dodge around the person in the middle to make it to the safety of the other end.

Staring down at you, with his only objective being to grab you, the guy in the middle would be fierce and quick. It would take skill and determination to run through the playground without bumping into someone else or being tagged. If you were tagged, then you had to go into the middle, and you would become that possessed person trying to grab the last of the runners. I used to do quite well. I was always one of the last people tagged. In the end there would only be a couple of us left being faced down by another ten people all wanting to grab us. The heart would beat hard, adrenaline flowing throughout the body, as you speedily accelerated forward. Flying across the playground, twisting and turning, weaving in and out, avoiding the touch of the guys in the middle.

This was one dangerous game, a game it was, but it was also real, fun and could be vicious. Many would fall, and fall hard. I remember there was a time when I had set off on my sprint, I was running hard and fast, but from the corner of my eyes I didn't notice an innocent bystander, watching us. My right foot fleetingly clipped theirs. Like a car wreck I was flung forward into the air and came crashing down onto my knees, hitting the concrete playground with force and momentum. I'm sure as my knees whacked into the concrete I bounced, then slid forward, scraping the skin straight off my knees. As I came to a stop, my whole body lunged forward to lie in a heap on the floor. The pain in my knees was unbearable and I could feel blood trickling down my legs.

Of course my stubbornness had started at a young age. I was about eight or nine then. I remained there on the floor for a moment in excruciating pain, but then the dinner whistle was blown. This is the point where we would all have to freeze. On the second whistle we would have to line up to go back inside. I somehow managed to stand, and stand still I did, blood dripping and trousers sticking to my skinless knees. It amazed me that my trousers had survived and weren't torn to shreds, but somehow they had.

With the second whistle blown I had to make it across the playground to line up. My god I could hardly move, with every step forward my trousers rubbed against the rawness on my knees. Perhaps this memory sticks in my head as clear as day because it hurt so damn much. But for the rest of the day I ignored it. It wasn't until I got home that night that I witnessed the devastation. Skin hanging off, blood stained legs, raw flesh with gravel mixed in. It looked like someone had taken a shot gun to my knees. How I made it through that day and carried on walking I do not know. Stubbornness of not being beaten I guess, something I must get a handle on!

Anyway, back to Gordon. As brutal as some of the games are, I think "British Bulldog" has now been banned in the playground, but I'm quite certain there are other games as brutal as ours once were. I didn't want him to miss out on his childhood. I wanted him to experience everything I had and so much more.

The waiting game was about to be over though. One fateful afternoon at work I received a call from my mother. It could have been about anything, but upon calling her back I learned that Rosemary had called and left a message for me to ring. I went out the back and out of the way of all the noise. This call was too important for it not to wait and phoned the number that had been left.

"Hello this is David Malarky. I've been left a message to ring you back."

"Hi David it's Rosemary at the EDS clinic. We have some news for you and you don't have to worry!"

"I don't have to worry? You mean its come back negative?"

"Yes David, we have just got the lab results back and thought it would be best to phone you first. We will send a write up to you, but it's okay. The test was negative, no mutation was found."

No mutation was found. Those words echoed around in my head for a minute, I felt my self becoming overwhelmed. A huge weight being taken off my shoulders, being released once again from the waiting game. There had been doubt in my mind and I was clutching at that hope, but finally this part of the journey was over. It was over. I could feel tears beginning to well up in my eyes, not tears of hurt of pain, but tears of so much joy.

"David we haven't rung Gordon's mother. We thought that it would be best coming from you. Is that okay if I leave it with you?"

"Yes. Yes of course, that's fine." My words were only just making it out and down the line and my voice began to crumble.

"Okay, well we shall look forward to seeing you soon at the next appointment then. Congratulations."

"Yes, yes thank you so much. Goodbye Rosemary."

The phone went dead. I stood there for a minute or two, silent, feeling the wind brush against my body, looking at my phone. Tears began to roll down my face. Every last minute of the last few weeks, all the fears and doubt being washed away. Gordon was in the clear. I stood there and I cried.

8

So here we are. Another part of the story has come and gone. Two negatives and and two positives. My hopes had been answered about Gordon, but the journey continued. When I came across Vascular Ehlers-Danlos I never fully realised the gravity of what it would lead to. All I was honed in on was the fact that it had tried to destroy me. I didn't really think of the consequences of my actions. Sure, knowing you have this can help a lot. My father had always had problems, I'd started to have problems, but Franny hadn't. Yes she did have medical problems but not in the major criteria. She had many issues with her stomach and with her joints however there was no possible way they could have been tied into something of this nature. Then there was my mother, strong willed, positive and so full of fight. An amazing woman who had stood right by my fathers side in his worst moments. Always there for him and always there for us. To be able to do that, to be able to stay sane, is a remarkable achievement in itself. But now not only had she my father to worry about, there was also myself, and possibly my sister. I had opened Pandora's box, and unleashed the savage beast, that not only causes physical carnage but also mental carnage.

Now here I will stray from the order of the time line again. The main reason being my brain is a little foggy and the order of the events is a little mixed up. Wouldn't yours be in this twisted tale? vEDS has a trait of causing brain fog. So I'm doing remarkably well to remember all the events that I have so far, I think.

But without further ado. Franny, my sister. Franny is a remarkable human being. As seems to be a trait in our family, she also has that "eye of the tiger," the "you can knock me down but I'm going to come back stronger" attitude. This obviously comes from our father on the physical side and our mother on the mental side. These are some of the best tools they have ever passed down to us, along with their loving caring nature of course.

Going back a few years now, I am going to tell you a short story about how remarkable Franny is. Are you keeping up, I hope so, but I do apologise for all the twists and turns. Now Franny was the passenger in a car accident. Said car had been travelling down a back road not far from the parent's, when the car left the road on a corner and ended up in a ditch late at night. She was trapped in the car, and without going into all the ins and outs, she did get hurt. Her hips and spine suffered the most. There was a lot of pain, a lot of bruising and her spine had been damaged. After this she couldn't walk far and was very immobile. Over the years to come she would have to learn to walk properly again. Through the

---

pain and the physio she fought, battling on and pushing herself. She could have sat back and let it beat her. But not Franny, she carried on and on and hasn't stopped. Of course it wasn't only the physical pain but also the mental fight. She also had to fight the problems of PTSD.

Within a few years she was still pushing. Fighting harder and harder every day. What she has been doing is remarkable. Franny found out about a charity called Brake. A road safety awareness organisation. She began to raise money for them to help victims of road traffic accidents. For her very first event she organised a quiz night at a local pub. It was hard work and she spent a lot of time organising. What followed was an amazing night with one hell of a turnout. The place was packed to the brim and money was raised. This in itself was fantastic. But she didn't want to stop there. Franny still wanted to do more to raise awareness. What she did next was amazing, all that fighting to learn to walk again, she went even further. This time, to raise more money and awareness for the charity, she decided to take on the challenge of walking up Snowdon. This was going to take some doing, hours of training, not an easy task. She did it though, then she did it again the following year at Scafell Pike and still she plans more; the next one being Ben Nevis. How about that, from being in the crash to walking up Ben Nevis. I am very proud of Franny. She has put her heart and soul into this and pushed herself far beyond where she has needed to, and been an inspiration and made a difference to so many people.

However as I said I had unleashed the beast from out of the box and the consequences of my actions were beginning to take form. Obviously with vEDS being a genetic trait I had just added to what she had to fight. I was about to change her life too. To bring in another monster. As I said before, Franny had problems, but didn't meet any of the major criteria. There was no major event that had been cause for concern. Franny had agreed to be tested. I don't think there was much choice either way really. If she hadn't have been tested, then she would still have thought about it. The only good that would come out of testing Franny would have been that the test was negative. This would have meant she could have gone on without having to worry about it. Without having to have the dark thoughts that lurk inside. The feeling as though something could happen at any time, the slightest twinge, the slightest pain frightening the life out of you wondering if an event was going to occur. Something or nothing, the fear of the unknown.

The usual process went on. Franny went to see the local GP, explained the situation and was referred to the genetics department. Within a few weeks the genetics department had seen her and given her the clinical diagnosis. Unlike Gordon they knew straight away by looking at her. This I thought would come to pass. I saw it in her as well, the bruising, the spontaneously bursting veins. It was all so familiar, just like my father and just like myself. Where there was doubt in my mind with Gordon, there was no doubt in my mind about Franny. I had been as certain that my brother was okay, as I had been as certain that my sister was not.

It was all too soon to realise it then. But there was a domino effect that was beginning to take place. Things were starting to build up which would start to break down the walls of my mind. Whilst the fight with Vascular Ehlers-Danlos is very physical and very real, there is another side to it that at first is not apparent. This thing has devastating effects and will challenge you in every way you can think of. It's an all out assault. When it's not hitting you physically, its attacking you from within the deepest corners of your mind.

So the clinical diagnosis they gave her was positive.

Obviously they still sent the blood samples away to confirm this, but again they came back positive. So now that's myself, my father and my sister all diagnosed with the same thing. Not the Hypertrophic Cardiomyopathy that we had all been checked for, but something far worse. Soon I will show you just how hard it strikes.

CHAPTER 5
THE ABANDONMENT OF HOPE

N ow the diagnoses were out of the way, well I say out of the way, but were they truly? On paper they may have been, but mentally there was still a long way to go in dealing with them. Remember that word that I didn't make up?

Denial
Anger
Bargaining
Depression
Acceptance.

This was a process that I have now seen myself go through. In some way, shape or form, we all do. Maybe we don't show it to anyone, but the battle inside our heads rages on. At this point in the journey I can now see I was in denial. Everything that had happened so far had been real, and true. But even so it still didn't feel real.

Christmas was drawing ever closer. It was now November 2013. Daily life was much the same. My health problems, well, there was nothing major going on. The dissection of the carotid still had it's lingering consequences, the migraines would still come and go. The lead weights, seemingly strapped to my legs, would randomly and suddenly reappear. Thunderstorms striking around inside my brain. Being set upon by sharp pains, making me unable to breathe or move for a few moments. Lots and lots of little things. They had never really affected me as much as they did since the dissection, but I had been beginning to get used to it over the past two years. It was becoming normal. Maybe I just started to notice them more because I had been diagnosed. Or perhaps my health had started to deteriorate a little more. If it was it would sound about right, remember my father was my age when his problems began. Perhaps I would be following this pattern.

But anyway moving forward, the next episode of "David Malarky's Life" was about to take place. This was set in my mind to be a big day, the day when we would find ourselves getting help. Today we would be visiting people who were going to keep us safe, keep us alive. I had a lot of hope resting on this. Yes I had already met perhaps the most knowledgeable person in the world on vEDS, but Gwen was a whole world away. All the way over the other side of the world in the gigantic land that is America. In truth I had only scraped the tip of the iceberg on the knowledge that she has, but she had given me the basic tools that I had needed to fight my way through the mist. Today though, I would be meeting people whom I would see on a regular basis. This was going to be the team that I would come to depend on, or so I thought. Our cardiovascular specialist, Dr Jayce Speed.

In their thoughtfulness the EDS clinic had set the appointment so that it was a double appointment with my father and I. We would both be going over at the same time to see Dr Speed. This was good, travelling from hospital to hospital takes its toll. Days organised off work, fuel costs, it all builds up and frankly you get a little sick of it. But they were thinking of us, it was only a couple of hours to get there, but it felt nice that they were thinking of us.

This time the appointment wasn't in the same building as the genetics clinic; the same hospital, but not the same building. This place was spread out all over. It was going to be quite a long day. On the agenda there was an MRI, an echo cardiogram and then to see the specialist himself. We had to be at the cardiology clinic at 9am to get prepared.

I will not bore you with the details of the journey there. Although I will say that it was early, so obviously it was time for the marvelous treat of sausage and egg Mcmuffin for breakfast. No road trip is complete without one remember! We used the same old multi-storey car park to park in, and at this time of morning the cars were beginning to line up to get in. Like the opening of a high profile concert, queueing to find a space to leave their mode of transport and embark on foot towards their destination. Moving along in line like ants with purpose.

This time instead of the long walk round to where the childrens ward resided, it was straight through the front doors. Have you ever seen "Superman"? Sure you have right, who hasn't? Well remember the Daily Planet building with the rotating double doors? Yes, there were rotating doors! I have always found the concept of rotating doors interesting. Constantly spinning, you have to time it right to get into the gap and follow the glass around until you get out through the doorway the other side. Sometimes you get the odd person who will try to fly through at the last available moment, barely making it in, and causing the motion sensor to stop the doors. The person inside, following the rotation is briefly trapped inside as the big wall of glass pauses in front of them. I wonder if anyone has ever been stuck in these before. They would perhaps make for an interesting human goldfish bowl!

So through the doors we went. Having no idea of where we had to be, well we did, the letter said cardiology, but where on earth was that! Signs, look for the signs ahead. Looking down the corridor past the waiting room, there were all manner of signs hanging from the ceiling. Brown, red, green, purple, blue, coloured signs everywhere. On the walls there were strips of colour flowing down the corridor to lead the way to each different department. Studying the signs, there was ours, green! The foyer was packed with people, like they had all just been herded in by a shepherd, standing in the middle of the floor, and all gazing up at those signs as if they were some sort of UFO flying through the sky. There were people everywhere. Seats were full, people reading papers, drinking coffee. Conversations of all types flowing through the air. It kind of reminded me of a food court at dinner time in a giant shopping centre.

Picking up the trail I walked in front of Howard. Five minutes to get to our first appointment, the MRI, and I didn't see any signs for the MRI scanning department so we followed the green lines to the cardiology department. Walking down big, wide corridors going further and deeper into the darker caverns. As we drew closer and closer there were fewer people. Gone were the crowds, now there was just the odd soul floating around, echoes of footsteps bouncing all around the white walls. But then we finally made it.

The darkness of the corridor gave way to a bright warm pink coloured waiting room. This place was huge. There were seats all over the place, doors going off here, there and everywhere. To the left as we came in, we were blinded by the light from the low morning sun piercing its way through the large ceiling to floor glass windows. In front of us there was a giant chest high counter, with admin staff sat behind it. Nurses were propped up at the end of it drinking their morning coffee, smiles on their faces as they talked of merriment.

Straight towards the desk we walked, and as I lay my letters on the counter I announced our presence.

"Good morning, I'm David Malarky and this is my father Howard. We have an appointment to see Dr Jayce Speed."

"Good morning David, Good morning Howard. Thank you for coming. Right lets have a look .. yes, yes, okay, right. First you will be seeing the nurse who will do an echo of your heart, then we will take you down for an MRI, and after you have been seen by one of the nurses to take some details we will take you through to see Dr Speed. Would you like to take a seat and someone will be with you shortly."

Rising from her seat, she raised her arm and pointed to all the hundreds of plastic blue chairs that lined the waiting room.

"Thank you."

With that I led the way over to the seating area, but before I even got the chance to sit down I was being approached.

"Good morning David," came the timid voice of an older lady who was shifting from the desk towards a door in front of us. "Would you like to follow me and we will take you through for an echo cardiogram, then we will do Howard."

I twisted round from my half sat half stood position and made my way through the door to a small room. In this small room was a bed with the obligatory white paper towel laid down on it, a chair at the end and next to the bed was the electrical machine that was the echo cardiogram. As the lady in the white ankle length lab coat came in she closed the door behind her.

"Could you strip off your top half for me and then lay down on the bed. I take it you have had this done before, but I'm going to hook you up and take a reading of your heart."

"Yes I know the score." I replied as I unbuttoned my shirt and proceeded to lie down.

"Right, lets get these pads on and get you hooked up. How was your journey?" She asked as she proceeded to stick me with the pads and then grab its oh so many leads, attaching them to the pads as she unravelled them all.

"It was all right thanks. Traffic wasn't too bad so it was quite an easy trip."

"That's good. Now if you lay still and breathe normally I'm just going to start taking the reading."

The nurse clicked a few buttons on the machine and it started to print off paper covered in a line that waved to the beat of my heart, ticking off little marks occasionally as it spewed it all out.

"There, that's it. We are done quick and painless, if you would like to get dressed again we shall get your dad sorted then we can take you down for the MRI.

Then she was back out of the door and beckoning Howard in. I took my seat for a few minutes and waited patiently for my father to reappear from the doorway. As he did the lady in the white coat beckoned us to follow her. Who she was I didn't know. She was moving swiftly and getting things done with grace. Obviously she had a busy day ahead of her. Leading us once again through the labyrinth we came to the MRI scanning department. This place seemed to be so much bigger than everywhere else. I was quite certain it never looked this big from the outside. It was like some sort of Tardis.

The unknown lady quickly spoke to the receptionist sat behind the desk and was soon ushering us through the waiting room and down yet another corridor.

"Howard if you would like to take a seat here, I will take David through and be back out for you in a minute."

I followed her into a changing room.

"David there is a locker there that you can put your

clothes in. If you would like to take this gown and put it on for me please. Can you also remove any jewellery that you are wearing."

Pulling back a curtain this bizarre lady almost pushed me behind it so that I could get changed. This woman wasn't messing around, she was most definitely on a mission to get things done and fast. I started to get myself undressed, the hairs on my body began to stand up as the coldness of the air touched my skin. As soon as I was ready she returned.

"Are you decent David?" came the voice from behind the curtain.

"Yep, I'm all ready for you." I said as I pulled the curtain back.

"Okay then follow me."

And off she went again, just around the corner and there it was. Stood there in the middle of the room. The giant white tube with the sliding bed protruding out of it's enclosed claustrophobic space. A machine similar to the one I began this story with. Obviously it wasn't the same machine as before. This was a different hospital, but you could be forgiven for thinking it was. It was identical in almost every way, even to where the window was carved into the wall where I'd seen the silhouettes before. Very familiar indeed.

As I approached the mechanised bed at the end of the scanner, there were two ladies standing there. One was pulling the paper towel across and the other wheeled across the machine that was going to pump that lovely dye through. This place was like a finely oiled machine. Each person had their purpose, they worked efficiently in unison to get the conveyor belt load of people through on time. I took my place on the bed, adjusted my gown slightly as not to expose myself to anyone.

"Good morning, lay back and carefully place your head in the restraint."

Slowly I began to lay back, shuffling myself up slightly. There was a fine gap that gave you a small margin of error to get your bonce in the head piece. I was becoming a pro at this by now and put my head to rest comfortably.

"Can I have your arm, so I can put a cannula in."A Spanish voice appeared behind me, reaching for my arm and taking it in her hands.

"There you go, I must warn you, it can be a little awkward to get in my veins." I replied nervously. I didn't like this part, people sticking things in me. It didn't hurt that much but was always an annoyance.

The lady looked at me and smiled "It's okay, I've had plenty of practice".

Which I'm sure she had. This was a busy place and I'm sure she was an expert at this judging by the way they all moved with much efficiency. She began the routine, tapping my veins as I clenched my fist to help in her search, tapping and tapping until she found one. Swiftly tearing open the wrapper on the cannula she moved it towards my vein.

"Quick pinch."

I felt it pierce my skin as she pushed down, through the first layer of my skin, moving it around slightly to line it up with my vein, into the vein, with another push.

"Are you okay?" as she halted for a moment.

"Yeah I'm all good." I replied, wincing a little as I felt her push again. Not painful, but an uncomfortable aching as she tried to push it in to place.

Then out it came again. She had found the vein but couldn't get it in. Swabbing the blood that trickled out of the pin prick hole she started to scan my arms with her eyes looking for another to try.

"Okay lets try the other arm, a little tricky aren't you?" smiling as if she was enjoying the challenge.

"I did say I was!" I smirked.

Now across to my right arm her attention was moved. Inside of the elbow she began to tap again, and again, as I clenched my fist to her aid her once again.

"I've got another, lets try this again, you still okay?"

"Yeah go for it."

For the minute I was finding it quite amusing that she was so confident she would get me first time. That would have been an almighty task.

"Right here we go, quick pinch."

She pushed down with another cannula, piercing the skin, positioning it around and deeper in she went as I felt it drag down, stopping momentarily as if it had come up against a concrete wall. Then with one final push I felt it give way and slide all the way in.

"There we go, got you!" As she started to secure it down with tape. "Right I'm just going to hook up the machine and make sure we have a good line. With that it began to pump, and as soon as she has pressed the button, I felt a sharp tearing pain in my arm where the cannula resided.

"Sugar."

She turned off the machine again and pulled the cannula back out quickly, pressing down hard on my arm with the cotton wool.

"Sorry that didn't work," she looked up at me a little puzzled, "Well I guess you did say you were awkward. Are you all right? It doesn't hurt too much does it?"

"A little but it's okay."

Of course it did hurt a little, my vein had just blown, there was going to be a nasty bruise there! As the Spanish lady kept pressing down on my right arm, another figure came walking up to me. Another nurse.

"Everything okay?" She questioned, looking at the Spanish dark haired lady still holding my arm.

"We seem to have a bit of an awkward one, his vein just blew, I can't get a good line in."

"Okay I'll give it a go if that's alright," Her gaze crossed from the Spanish nurse to myself and then down my left arm where the first attempt had taken place, "Are you on blood thinners?"

Looking at my arm I replied, "Yes, I had a stroke." There was blood trickling out from that pinpoint hole, all the way down my arm and had dripped on the floor. I hadn't noticed this before, as I had been a little distracted.

"Here let me just wipe this off."

She took my left arm and proceeded to wipe the blood off.

"Now, lets have a look on this arm again." Her eyes began scanning up and down, as she turned her attention to my left wrist. "This one looks good."

I now had two nurses by my side. The Spanish lady had stopped putting pressure on my arm and moved back a little and was watching. I could see a bruise forming on my right arm already.

"Right, quick pinch." The new nurse said as another cannula broke through that first layer of skin. For a moment she jolted back and forwards, pushing it in, then back out and in again. I winced as I felt her push it in, then as soon as it was in, there it was again, another sharp tearing pain.

"Damn, that ones blown, I didn't even get it in properly, what's wrong with you?" she said a little confused.

"I have Vascular Ehlers-Danlos Syndrome."

"What's that?"

"It's a connective tissue disorder. We have weak veins and arteries, I thought you knew about this?"

"Oh right, no never heard of it."

I found that very bizarre. I thought I was in the place of knowledge. I thought these people knew what was wrong with me. Surely she must have known?

"Well I think I'll just go and get a doctor to come and have a look if that's okay?"

"Yeah, okay."

This was beginning to frustrate me a little. Being prodded and poked is bad enough. But being prodded and poked by people who were supposed to know what vEDS was, was making me a little uncomfortable.

Within a couple of minutes the nurse came back with another lady by her side. This one looked a little smarter, a doctor I could only presume. She walked up to me and hardly acknowledged me. Taking my arms she scanned up and down. Then she spoke.

"What do you have?" she asked.

"Vascular Ehlers-Danlos Syndrome." I replied a little shortly without my normal humorous tone.

"Right, I don't know what that is, but I take it it's something to do with your veins?"

"Yes it is, the collagen is faulty."

My faith in this place was deteriorating. I thought people here knew about this. I thought they had at least heard the name before even if they didn't know the ins and outs of it.

The doctor pulled up my left hand.

"Right lets try by the thumb. I can see the veins clearly, I was thinking of getting an ultrasound machine down here but I don't think we will need it as that doesn't seem to be a problem."

She began tapping away at my vein again until it rose in all its glory.

"Okay, this might pinch a little more but is usually a good one."

In went the next cannula through the first layer of skin and once more puncturing another vein. Pushing and moving around again, pulling at the skin as it went, a deep aching pain where the cannula was being pushed in and out, she got in the vein, pushed and there it was.

"Ahh" I let out a sigh as I felt the searing pain as the vein popped.

Removing the cannula and pressing down to stop the bleeding the doctor apologised. I simply nodded in acknowledgement. She was young, maybe it was inexperience. My right arm where the first vein had popped was itching a little, my left arm where the second vein had popped had begun to itch. The first one on my left arm just ached.

"Right this is strange, well I'm afraid I have to go, I've got a meeting, you'll just have to call Dr Mertle down to have a look. Get her to try those two on the right arm." She ordered as she left the room.

"We're sorry about this David, I'll get Dr Mertle one of the senior doctors to have a look. It looks like you're going to have a few bruises I'm afraid. Would you mind following me and we will sit you in another room while we scan someone else?"

I stood and followed the Spanish nurse back out of the room. She took me into another room just behind the MRI room. There were cupboards all around with a wheelchair in the middle of the floor. I was being placed into some sort of giant walk in store cupboard.

I sat there as the nurse left. She had promised she would be as quick as she could. In my gown I sat, my arms beginning to ache from being prodded and poked. I ran my hands up and down my arms not only to comfort the aching but it was bloody freezing in there. It was November and there was no heating in the room and I was in a thin ass hospital gown. I was a little shocked with what was happening. From out the corridor I could faintly hear the voices of two nurses talking.

"Yeah it's weird, every time we get a cannula in his veins just burst, I've not seen anything like it." came a whisper.

Me, they were talking about me. The freak who keeps

exploding. When I came out this morning I wasn't expecting anything like this. In fact quite the opposite. I was expecting answers. I was expecting people who knew, who could help me. This was the turning point. It was now becoming real. Sitting there, alone, in a damn glorified storage cupboard. People whispering about me in the background in amazement of this person with veins that are exploding. But I'd had this done before without any problems, had I suddenly become weaker, was I getting weaker?

"I have Vascular Ehlers-Danlos Syndrome. Shit."

Everything that had happened in the past couple of years was real. It wasn't some sort of nightmare that I was going to wake up from. This was it, this is my life. I have Vascular Ehlers-Danlos Syndrome!

Eventually another doctor came down. She knelt down in front of me and must have seen the sorrow that had swept across my face with my realisation.

"Hi David I'm - are you .. okay?" she looked at me taking my hands in hers and, sliding her hands up and down my arms, "you're cold!"

"Yeah, I'm fine, I think, just want to get this done now and get out of here." I replied quietly, not really looking her in the eyes.

"Okay David, lets have a look. There's a couple more veins I can try on your right arm and the final one on the top of your right hand. We will go for the one midway down your arm first."

The same usual routine ensued, tapping prodding, poking and piercing. As soon as it was in, the sharp tearing pain returned, followed by itching. My arms we starting to become covered, I was going to be black and blue for days, even the first hit on my left arm that hadn't popped. Onwards to the one on the top of my right hand. Again exactly the same. In, pop, in pop! Nothing was working, my veins were too weak to even hold the simplest thing such as a cannula.

"I'm sorry David, I'm going to stop now. We've had way too many attempts. We have never seen anything like this before. I will ring your doctor and see if we can do the MRI without the dye."

With that she left me sat in the room with my own thoughts again. My own thoughts of realising that my body is broken. I'm broken, I really am broken! Humpty Dumpty fell off a wall and broke, I didn't need even need to fall. The weight that had once been lifted off my shoulders with Gordon getting the all clear was starting to come back. I could feel myself slipping into a dark place.

A few moments later the original Spanish nurse returned. As she walked back in she smiled at me, I didn't smile back. They had been talking about me like I was some kind of freak. Of course I was. I was different, I'm not like the others.

"Right David, we have the all clear, we are going to go ahead with the scan without the dye. It's not the best solution but it will still give an indication of what they are looking for."

What were they looking for you ask? Well they were looking for aneurysms or any other foreseeable events to do with my arteries.

I was taken back through and placed in the cocoon. Left there for another forty minutes, whilst it buzzed and banged and whirred liked the tape loading of the Commodore 64. Left there, in the cold gown, motionless, holding my breath as they scanned me over and over. The occasional radio chatter through the headset giving me instructions of when to breathe and when not to. Repeatedly, asking me if I was okay. No, I was not okay. My arms ached. I was broken beyond repair. My foundations, threatening to collapse at any given moment, and not a damn thing I nor anyone could do about it. Alone in a world where no one cares.

2

So the scan was done, I had got dressed. I had spoken to myself whilst in there, and told myself it didn't matter. We are about to see the best this country has to offer. There was still hope, we can be helped and they will help.

As we were led back down the twisty catacombs my father turned to me.

"You were along time in there, what happened?"

"They couldn't get a cannula in."

"What do you mean? Mine was in first time." he answered, looking puzzled.

"Every time they got one in the vein would burst. I'll show you later, my arms are really sore."

I rubbed my arms up and down as we walked. Then we were back in the waiting room. But we carried on straight through out to another corridor, which had more seats lining it, with doors all the way down, more like being back at the local doctor's surgery. We didn't even get to sit down when a tall man, standing around 6ft 2, I'm useless with guessing heights, but he was tall, came towards us.

"Good Morning David, Good morning Howard, I'm Dr Jayce Speed, would you like to come in?"

Holding out his arm he motioned to a room on our right. There was a desk directly in front against a wall, sat to the left of that were Rosemary and Dr Gazelle Banger whom we had obviously met before. Two chairs were laid out in front of the desk. Closing the door Dr Jayce moved passed us and sat down behind his desk.

"Please sit down," he said, and that we did.

Gazelle in her quiet soft voice smiled at us, "Hello David and Howard, how are you both doing?"

"Good thanks" said Howard.

"Yeah awesome" I said, trying to hide the sarcasm a little. I wasn't quite so pissed off now, but I was still a little disappointed.

Rosemary didn't say anything, she just looked up from her notepad and smiled at us both.

"Well I'm Dr Speed and I'm a vascular consultant. You already know these guys from seeing them previously. We are all here today because I'm going to be overseeing you both and Gazelle is here to advise on the EDS side of things. I'll be honest, I have not seen many patients with vascular type, so Gazelle is my expert in that."

Silently in my head, I let out a little "hmmm," I thought this guy was a vEDS specialist.

"As you know, Ehlers-Danlos is a connective tissue disorder, and in the vascular type it involves a mutation of the COL3A1 gene which is found mainly in the hollow organs, the veins and the arteries. Collagen is basically like the glue that holds us together. Whilst you produce enough collagen, it is faulty and in essence means that it doesn't stick together as well as it should. Whilst there isn't any cure, our aim is to monitor the vascular system, look out for any aneurysms."

My father broke into words, "The aneurysms, what do you do if you find any?"

"If we find any, we take measurements to see how large they are and monitor them to see if they grow."

"And if they grow?" my father replied.

"If they grow, it depends on where they are as to whether we do anything. With vEDS being what it is we tend to advise away from any sort of invasive procedure, unless it's a very life threatening problem. The reason is of course with the arterial walls being weak, they tear and can often make the problems worse leading to low survival rates for surgery."

"Well if you find any in me I'd rather not know thanks."

"So what your saying is you don't really do anything?" I asked just to be clear.

"We can, but it would have to be carefully done, by a specialist vascular surgeon. It's very risky. Now Howard, I understand you were diagnosed with Hypertrophic Cardiomyopathy?" he turned his attention solely to my father.

"That's right. When I was David's age I had my first heart attack and they diagnosed me with that, and since then I've numerous heart attacks and angina attacks."

"Do you know what type of heart attacks they were?"

"No, no-one's ever told me, I just thought a heart attack was a heart attack."

"Well a heart attack can also be caused by a tear in the artery, so I'm wondering whether this could have accounted for some of your vascular events. I'm not saying that the HCM doesn't add to it but I would be more inclined to think that vEDS is more the cause of the pain you experience."

"Oh right well I don't know, they just said that's what I've got and left it at that really. The vEDS thing I don't really know a lot about apart from what David found out as no one has ever mentioned it before."

"Yes David, I've heard it was you that found it? How did you manage that with it being so rare?" Shifting his gaze over to me he looked a little intrigued.

"If I'm honest, after the dissection I was getting a little annoyed. I was being passed from pillar to post. No-one was coming up with any answers. My neurologist just kept telling me how lucky I was and how bizarre it was for this to happen without any trauma. I had a little bit of time on my hands, so I started looking through Google once I knew what had actually happened. It wasn't the easiest of things. I looked through case studies and in one I came across a link to EDS. I clicked it and started reading, as I got into it I found vascular type. Going off my problems and family history I started to piece it together."

Nodding his head, "Well that's quite remarkable really. I see you have been a few places, even down to London."

"Yeah a big waste of time that was. I was sent there and the guy hadn't even seen any of my notes or my scan results, just told me to stick to my local neurologist."

"Okay well you're here now, that's the main thing. So we will try and take care of you. So medication wise. Howard, I'm leaving yours as they are. I've looked down the long list and I can't really see a point in changing any of it at this late stage. There are some items that I might think about taking you off, you've already got a beta blocker in there, so I'd rather not introduce anything else to upset the balance. David now I see you're on a blood thinner which is obviously for the stroke?"

"Yeah. Would it be best to come off that? I have also been told to get onto Celiprolil?"

"Celilprolil, who's told you this?"

Now he really was interested.

"Well, long story short I have been in contact with a vEDS specialist in America. Gwen Patroni. She works at a medical company and is carrying out research into vEDS. She mentioned that in France they had trialled a small research program with this Celiprolil. The results weren't conclusive but looked promising."

"You seem to know what you talking about David. Have you heard of this Gazelle?"

He shifted his gaze across to Gazelle. So far she hadn't really said a lot, just sitting listening in the background taking notes with Rosemary. She began to shake her head.

"No, it's not something I've heard about if I'm honest."

"Right, well okay we can have a look into that. The blood thinners, you are quite right, you don't really want to be on them with having vEDS" Of course I already knew this.

"Although we need to find out more about this stroke. Did they say whether it was caused by the dissection?"

"No they didn't tell me anything like that. They think it might be an older occurrence, separate to the dissection but they were more focused on the dissection itself."

"Okay. I'll write to your neurologist and get his opinion. The problem with the blood thinner is that if you have an arterial rupture they could make it worse. The bleed will be greater. So we are going to have to weigh up which is better."

"A catch 22 situation then? The lesser of two evils?"

"Yes more or less I'm afraid. We will decide that when we find out. I will also write to your doctor so he can decide which way he wants to go when we have the results." He looked backwards and forwards at my father and myself. "Have either of you got any more questions?"

"Yes I have," said Howard, "I have kidney stones which they have tried to laser out before, the pain they cause me is getting unbearable and I want them cut out. I'm seeing a specialist at my local hospital to try and get him to do it but he's being evasive. Would you recommend it?"

"Well no not really. You've got to realise that any operation is dangerous and can create complications. You have to take a step back and see if the risk outweighs the problems."

"I'm adamant, I want these out, I can't keep going on

like this. No pain killers touch it any more."

"Hmm. What do you think Gazelle, any experience with anything like this?"

Gazelle shook her head again, "Sorry but we just don't know. As you say it's risky, and we just don't have any figures. Any operation is potentially life threatening. I don't think anybody would be willing do it. Sorry."

"It really needs to be done. I want them out, I don't care." said my father with a hint of desperation.

Dr Speed looked back at my father again, "Well if you really think it is worth the risk of potentially not waking up then we can talk about it. Talk to your specialist, if he needs to, then he can talk to me. If he will do it and you do decide to go ahead, then they must have a vascular surgeon on hand, it's imperative. All right any more questions?"

"Not really" I said, "I don't think at the minute there is. We know the basics I suppose. Although I do sometimes get these sharp random pains that hurt that much I cant move or breathe. They are usually just off the centre of my chest, to the lower left of my stomach and just under my right breast and usually last around 20 minutes."

"Anything like that and you should really get it checked. It's probably nothing, but I cannot stress how important it is. If it's a vascular event that is happening, the sooner it gets checked out the better the chances are."

"Okay, but how long do you leave it before getting worried?"

"That's a good question but not one that can be answered really. If you are worried, then get checked and make sure you have your emergency info with you."

Dr Speed glanced at us both and smiled. "If there is nothing else I'd just like to have a quick physical look at you both if I may? Howard, you first."

Dr Speed got up from behind his desk and led my father into a back room. While they were gone Gazelle began quizzing me on how I had come to meet this American doctor. I told her the story of how I had strangely met Pink Lily. Then of how we had been looking into things and stumbled across Gwen. I told them briefly the tale of how I had come to Skype her and had signed up for the research. They seemed generally impressed with this.

After a few minutes passed by, my father reappeared and Dr Speed's voice bellowed out from the room beyond, "Would you like to come through now David."

I got up and went through. "Would you like to take a seat on the end of the bed for me, and could you roll up your sleeves, unbutton your shirt and roll up your trousers?"

I did this and Dr Speed began to examine me. Looking at my over flexible fingertips, the stretchy skin on my elbows and the translucent skin around my chest and neck. He saw my bruised arms where I had been pricked and prodded.

"This doesn't look too good, what happened?"

"They couldn't get a cannula in, I thought you knew?"

"No not at all. Why couldn't they get one in? That's going to be a right mess."

"Every time they managed to get it in, the vein would blow."

"Oh no. I'm sorry, that's really bad. Well if they have done it without the dye it should be all right, but we may have to do it again."

"No I don't think so, not after that. There were a lot of people trying, two nurses and two doctors. There's no way I'm going through that again."

"We will see how we get on. So what other problems do you have on a daily basis?"

"Well I suppose I get fatigued quite easily. I also have

problems with my muscles. If I run then my thigh muscles don't last long and feel like they are going to tear. It also feels like that sometimes when I walk upstairs. Its often that painful that I have to walk up sideways. Apart from that, there's the migraines I have had since the start of the dissection, which I take it are a product of the dissection. I used to have them when I was a teenager, but grew out of them. I struggle to sleep at night, sometimes can take up to four hours of laying there and no matter how much or how little sleep I get I always struggle to wake up in the morning."

"You certainly seem to have been doing your research. That's good because I'm afraid the reality is you have to be your own doctor so to speak. You have to learn to get to know your body. When we are trained, EDS isn't really covered much so not many people will know about it, and you will probably be looking at the same articles documented that we use. Even though EDS has been around for years, it has been relatively unexplored. Vascular in particular is even worse, there's probably a lot more people out there, but its often the case they don't get diagnosed until it's too late."

"That's a pretty sad scenario. I was really hoping it wasn't going to be this and I would be laughed at, but here we are."

"You've done a good job. The important thing to remember is that knowing gives you a chance. As horrible and scary as it can be the odds are better now than if you did not know."

Dr Speed's voice was frank and sympathetic, he didn't know a great deal but he also didn't try to make out that he did.

"Okay right. David, that's it we are done."

And that was it, we were done. Obviously we said our thank yous and goodbyes. I did appreciate they had taken the time to see us. I couldn't help but feel disappointed though. The cold hard truth was that I hadn't learned anything new. I already knew everything that had been said. In fact I was probably starting to learn more than they had. Okay, so I wasn't a doctor, I didn't know all the fancy words and terminology for everything.

"You have to be your own doctor."

I was beginning to hear this a lot. You're faced with a life threatening illness and you hear those words. What is that? Why is that? There should be someone looking after us, curing us. We had entered an unwinnable battle. Nobody knew what was going to happen to us, nobody knew how to stop it. Fighting every day of our lives to stay alive. And that's what this is about. Everyday we face the unthinkable. We have been and we are still fighting to stay alive. Wondering if the next pain is going to be the last pain. Is this what knowing is about? Am I really this broken that I can't be fixed? It appears so. This was the reality of the situation. We are not about to be given a chance to be cured. We can't have just one fight against it, this thing was going to beat us down and keep attacking. There wasn't anything that could stop this, and now I was beginning to realise how very real this had become. Hope was fading a little. They couldn't even complete the simplest task of putting a cannula into my veins. Was it really possible that they were becoming weaker? I can't believe that there is no one that is going to come and save us. In this day and age of medical advancements and there is nothing. It makes no sense.

3

Before we go on, I'm going to divert your attention away, as I think this little incident plays a big part in developing understanding. As I sit here and write this in the present day, November 2014, I was last night reminded of the true horrors that we face. I will try not to keep you here too long and will get straight to the point.

I haven't been well for the past couple of days. Just the usual visual disturbances, pain in the head, whether it be your average migraine or the lingering results of the dissected carotid I do not know. It is what it is. With my new found ability of swallowing my pride to make sure I look after myself I have taken a couple of days off work.

Last night I went to bed, feeling quite okay with plans to resume work the next day. I was lying watching a couple of episodes of Homeland, nicely relaxed. Turning the TV off, I embarked on the mission of trying to get to sleep. Within about half an hour I was getting there, halfway to nodding off. Out of nowhere I was hit by a severe onset of a sharp tearing pain on my right hand side, halfway up the rib cage. Now I have had pains like this before, however this was a little more intense. I tried to move a little, my mobile phone was close, but I couldn't move.

Every time I tried to move even just an inch there would be an horrendously sharp pain. Imagine a knife, stuck inside you, then when you move, the knife takes a deep cut. The more you move, the more it rips through you. I truly couldn't move, not only in fear of something seriously going wrong, but it hurt that much. As I took breaths in there was exactly the same thing, I had to make shallow controlled breaths in order for whatever it was not to be ripped to shreds.

For around thirty minutes I lay there. Trapped. There was nothing I could do. You might think I'm exaggerating, after all us males do have a tendency to exaggerate right? No, I promise you, no exaggeration. My own body had me pinned down. I always have my phone close to hand, as this is my lifeline, for moments just like this. The phone was on the bedside table, well within reaching distance, but it wasn't, because in that instant there was nothing I could do. It was impossible to move at all. I was completely alone with only my thoughts to keep me company.

What goes through your head when this happens? Well you try to rationalise it, try to convince yourself that it is nothing serious. You don't really know whether it is or not. Is it muscle damage, is it lung problems, is it a small tear, is it a major tear? Time ticks by and still the pain continues, still trapped. Panic begins to kick in, it's not stopping. Is it getting worse, is it going to stop? Is this the one? Is this what my life accumulates to? Laying here alone in my bed unable to move, unable to seek help. The uncertainty that you try so hard to keep at bay and keep the faith that everything is going to be okay, but you know there is a very real possibility that this is the end!

Even if I could have reached my phone, if I could have called someone, there were still two flights of stairs to battle down to get the front door unlocked. Would I have made it without falling down the stairs? Would I have been able to get that far? These are the thoughts you have to deal with, have to try to rationalise with and try to keep calm. Your life hangs in the balance and you feel fear.

Luckily as soon as the pain had come, it had gone. Not a single trace left. I slowly got up, picked my phone up and went downstairs to get a glass of water. Now if there had been any sort of pain left I would have gone straight to Accident and Emergency. But I rationalised it. I figured that it couldn't have been anything too serious, as if it was then surely it would have left its mark. But it didn't, nothing, as though I had imagined it. I hadn't of course, it was very real. Panic over thank the stars, but I would in the morning call my local doctor and get it investigated further.

The morning came and I rang my local surgery, but this was to no avail. No appointments, they told me to ring back this evening after 6:30pm. I rang again and still the same, no appointments. I rang the next morning and the next but still no appointments. All they would offer me was an appointment in two weeks' time. I asked if they could get a doctor to call me back, to be answered with a blunt "No". Now, I don't like making too much of a fuss, but after the third day I was getting a little annoyed, so I said to the receptionist that I had a life threatening condition and really needed to see or speak to a doctor. Again I was met with a brick wall. The receptionist simply said that if it was life threatening then I should visit the Accident and Emergency. Understandable on their side really, but of course I knew by now that it wasn't life threatening, I hadn't had the pain as severely again, although there was a niggle that had kept on coming back. All I wanted was to get it checked out. But no, this wasn't happening.

After a week of trying I finally got through and got an appointment, not with my regular doctor whom I would have preferred, but with another one. At least this was something and I could perhaps get to the bottom of the source of the pain. How wrong could I have been.

It was a late appointment so I left work early that day. I had given myself plenty of time to get to the doctors as the drive was about an hour away. What was about to happen was going to leave me in disbelief and leave me more frustrated than I had ever been. Upon pulling into the car park it was fairly empty. The sun had set and given way to the darkness of the night. The light from the street lights reflected off the damp ground. As I made my way across the car park to the big automatic surgery doors, I walked through, catching my shoulders between the doors as I went. It appeared that that they didn't open as fast as I wanted to walk. The surgery was quite empty. A queue of people were lined up at the receptionists desk, but there was no one sat down in the waiting area. It was looking like they were getting ready to close. To the automated check in machine I strode, entering my initials and my date of birth, at which the machine would react and tell me go and take a seat upstairs and wait until Dr Dolittle called me.

As I sat there in the upstairs corridor, much like the downstairs one I had been in so many times before, my chest began to flutter a little. Maybe nerves, maybe anxiety, making me feel a little light headed. Going to the doctors always seemed to do this, no matter had many times I had been or wherever I'd been, I would always feel nervous. I guess it was something to do with the fact that I just hated anything medical. Whether I will ever get used to it or not, I do not know. However within a few minutes a door down the corridor opened.

"David Malarky please!"

This was one voice that couldn't be missed, it bellowed down the hall reverberating around my ear drums. This chap was huge, not in an overweight type of way but he was tall, standing well over 6ft, in my mind I would possibly even go as far as saying he was getting on for 7ft. I had never seen him before, a man of South African descent, or Caribbean maybe? I'm not that great with this type of guess work.

As I rose from my seat I made my way down the corridor towards the giant as he ushered me into his room.

"Good afternoon, and what can we do for you today?"

"Hello. I've been having this pain that I would like looking at, I don't think its anything too serious but I would like to get it checked out. Have you seen my notes?"

"No I haven't, but what type of pain is it?"

"Well I don't have it right at this minute but it started last week. This is the first time I have been able to get in to see anyone."

"Okay, tell me more."

"I was laid in bed and I had a sudden severe onset of sharp localised pain right here." I moved my hand and indicated a line right across where the pain had been, half way up my rib cage on the right hand side of my body.

"Right okay. And you don't have the pain any more?"

"No not at this minute, but it comes and goes, it's not come back anywhere near as bad as the other night. I couldn't move when I had it then. I would have gone to Accident and Emergency if I had been able to, but after thirty minutes or so it completely disappeared without a trace. You really should look at my notes in fact .. here."

As I said this I pulled out my wallet and gave Dr Doolittle the folded piece of paper with the emergency medical info on it. He begin reading.

"Vascular Ehlers-Danlos Syndrome, what is this?"

"Well -" but he cut me off.

"It's okay. I'm thinking out loud. I'll read."

There was silence as he began to read the paper laid out before him, his facial expressions turning to panic and fear in what he was digesting:

Medical Alert information for Vascular Ehlers-Danlos Syndrome

Vascular Ethlers-Danlos syndrome (vEDS) is a life threatening connective tissue disorder that affects all tissues, arteries and internal organs making them extremely fragile.

vEDS patients are at risk of sudden arterial or organ

rupture. This can occur at any age. Mid-size arteries are commonly involved.

Patients' concerns should be taken seriously and any reports of pain need full and immediate investigations

<u>Presenting symptoms</u>

Arterial or intestinal rupture commonly present as sudden acute abdominal, chest or pelvic pain, that can be diffuse or localised.

Cerebral arterial rupture may present with altered mental status and be mistaken for drug or alcohol use.

Redness, pain and prominence of one or both eyes and the sound of pulsations in the head can be manifestations of a carotid-cavernous fistula.

Vascular dissection and rupture or bleeding can be subtle in presentation, therefore a lower threshold for investigations and imaging is indicated.

<u>Management guidance</u>

The fragility of all tissues means that invasive procedures should be avoided in vEDS where possible.

All members of the medical team should be aware of the potential risk for greater than usual harm.

•Immediate investigation by MRI or CT scan should be performed.

•Use non-invasive techniques only, avoiding stress and tension on skin, organs and vessels during physical examination.

•Avoid angiography, enema and endoscopies.

•Avoid intramuscular or subcutaneous haematoma and bruising.

•Central lines should be placed only with ultrasound guidance to avoid inadvertent arterial injuries.

•Bleeding in the body wall or cavity should be managed conservatively with transfusion and support.

Emergency Surgery

Surgical risks are higher for vEDS patients. The threshold for intervention should be higher. All conservative management options should be carefully considered before surgery.

The primary indication for surgical intervention is life threatening ruptured arterial complications.

• A vascular surgeon should be present during surgery.

• The anaesthetist should be aware of fragile mucus membranes when intubating.

• Self retaining retractors should be used carefully, excessive retraction leads to multiple tissue tears and haematomas.

• Tissues are fragile and do not hold sutures well.

~Created by the Ehlers-Danlos Syndrome National Diagnostic Service

"Oh my gosh what is this? This is terrible, oh my

word."

A look of bewilderment entered his face.

"Arterial dissection. Oh no, oh my gosh. This is bad, MRI scan, CT scan, intestinal rupture? Oh my word what are you doing here?"

"Well like I said, I have spoken to the EDS clinic and they have said it would be best to come and check it out. I don't think it's anything serious as if it was I would have known about it by now."

He looked at me in amazement. "This is serious, dissection?"

"Yes, a couple of years ago I had a dissection of the carotid artery."

"What? Carotid dissection, no?"

"Yes its in my notes."

With that he looked up at the computer screen before me and started flicking through. He stopped on a letter of correspondence stating the finding of my MRI scan.

"Oh my gosh, you've had a right internal carotid dissection?"

"Yes I did, a couple of years ago. It was spontaneous."

"You can't be here, what are you doing to me? We can't help you!"

With that I burst out with a laugh, of disbelief.

"What do you mean? Like I said I don't think its serious, but I would like to find out what it is, or at least get some idea of what it could be."

"We can't help you. There's nothing we can do, you're complicated, you could have another dissection, you can't be here, you should have gone to Accident and Emergency, this is serious stuff."

"Well I know it's a serious condition but I don't think this event is serious."

"It doesn't matter, this is dangerous stuff."

I was beginning to feel like I was talking to a brick wall. I knew this wasn't some sort of serious event and all I wanted was for him to take a look and advise me on what it could be. I'm not a doctor and I didn't know what it was, but if it had been serious then by now I would have been in trouble.

"Okay look, we need to check your blood pressure and listen to your chest. Unbutton your shirt, please."

As I started to unbutton my shirt he reached for his stethoscope and began to place its coldness on my chest. As I breathed in and out he listened in various places.

"Right that seems okay. Now come and lay down over here."

Dr Doolittle raised his arms and pointed to the bed that was on the opposite side of the room.

"Okay lie down."

As I laid there the doctor began feeling around me looking for points of pain, but there was nothing. Everything felt quite all right.

"Yes, that seems okay. Now take a seat again."

Once again I moved back over to my chair and sat down. There was another moment of silence as the doctor scanned through my notes further and looked at the leaflet I had handed him.

"A stroke as well, this is crazy? I don't know what you want me to do? Have I taken your blood pressure, we need to take your blood pressure."

"No you haven't."

Was he panicking, this tall statue of a man, had I scared him that much and he was fearful of the patient that he had sat before him?

"Okay let's take your blood pressure."

Why was he looking to me for answers? With that he placed the cuff of the blood pressure monitor around my arm. As it blew up I could feel it getting tighter and tighter around me. Pins and needles started to fill my fingers as it gripped me and cut off the blood supply.

"Yes that's okay I think, I think its okay, Let me look

at your eyes."

I looked at him straight in the eyes, and I saw confusion. Panic, even.

"They look okay, that's good, do you have the pain now?"

"No not at all. As I said it's been coming and going."

"Well I don't think it's anything serious, I think you're okay, but you should have gone to Accident and Emergency, there is nothing I can do for you."

"I know it's nothing serious, that's why I came here and not A and E, because I wanted to see what it could be." I replied again with frustration and annoyance filling my voice.

"I need a copy of this leaflet, we need to keep one," he said as he picked up the phone and called down to reception to tell them I was coming down to have it photocopied and placed with my notes.

When he put the phone down he went back to the computer and started filling in more details. I saw that on there it only stated "Ehlers-Danlos Syndrome" and no mention of vascular type which he was now changing this to. He also typed that the patient was reassured what to do in an emergency situation. Then he turned his attention back to myself.

"Look, if it happens again then you must go to Accident and Emergency, it is very important."

"Well I know that, but like I said I know it's not serious and just want some help, what do you think it could be?"

"It's the vEDS. It could have been a bleed, it will have been the vEDS. If it happens again, A and E. You must. Now before you leave you must get this copied at reception."

And that was it. That was what the appointment had amounted to. This massive man and become small and scared I think. He'd panicked at what he had seen and wasn't going to give me any help apart from telling me to go to hospital. In reality, the pain could have been something as simple as muscle pain, a gall bladder problem, or some sort of issue with a nerve. It could have been any number of things, but this doctor had just shipped me out without wanting to help me get to the bottom of it. It was complete and utter madness. The whole experience shocked me, never had I seen anyone act this way. But it is was it is, this is just the way things are. Welcome to a life with being diagnosed with Vascular Ehlers-Danlos Syndrome. The saying has never been truer:

"You have to be your own doctor"

In hindsight, I don't really think any other doctor's reaction would have been that different, maybe slightly different in the way they composed themselves. But at the end of the day, in reality, there wasn't a great deal he would have been able to do for me. He was right really. I should have gone to A and E, closer to the time.

4

Back to the past then. Back to November 2013 after the appointment that was meant to be full of greatness. This was supposed to a turning point, a turning point for the better. However it wasn't. That appointment was the end result of a lot of different events. Everything had steered us in that direction towards the place that I hoped would give us answers. It was supposed to end here. Not end here, but at least be the end of looking after ourselves. This was supposed to be a time where we could breathe a sigh of relief and have a little confidence that everything would be okay. It was far from this though. What came from that appointment was the opposite. It was the realisation that we were on our own. This I would not accept easily. There had to be something out there that could save us. I still clung to hope, after all, there was still research that I was taking part in.

As I said to you before, I would talk about hope. That special four letter word that carries so much weight with it. If you have hope then you can keep moving forward, you can keep battling on against everything. But what happens when hope begins to fade? The light that was shining so brightly, slowly letting a darkness consume you. Well I have been toying with the question of whether I should take you down this road. Am I really ready to let you see deep inside of my soul? Maybe not. But if I'm to tell the story right then I have to take you to the places I have been. Whatever you think of me now I do not know. Whatever you will think of me when all this is over I do not know. As we delve down this path, please remember this is not about sympathy. This is about so much more than that. This is no longer about me, this is no longer about my family, now there is a bigger picture, a bigger purpose. Whatever has happened in my life, what ever will happen from now on I want it all to have meaning. And so with that it mind, I'm taking you to a place where I didn't want to go. Follow me.

"You have to be your own doctor"

After the appointment with Dr Speed I was beginning to realise that Vascular Ehlers-Danlos was worse than I initially thought. Due to the lack of knowledge, the lack of people diagnosed was not great. I thought being diagnosed would help us all, but I was starting to feel like it wouldn't. I was starting to wish I had never pursued this. There was a guilt starting to build up inside of me. What I had actually done was starting to weigh down on me. My sister had already been fighting her many battles and now here I was giving her another one. She was okay. There's a chance that she always would be, but now I had brought this monster into her life. Yes it gave answers to some of the little things, but it was the mental side I had brought to her doorstep.

80% of people by the age of 40 have a major event.

Now she had to worry about this. These figures on paper laid out to scare the life out of you.

Average lifespan of a person with vEDS: 52 years

Okay so it's an average figure, people either side, young and old alike. My father was nearly sixty. But did it matter? vEDS didn't follow a pattern. It just attacked you when it felt like it. It would beat you down everyday, and when it had toyed with you enough it would kill you. That is one thing that is certain. Vascular Ehlers-Danlos is a cold blooded killer.

To show you just how horrible it can be, I will tell you what I found. One night, when I was searching through the internet I came across a newspaper article. It was the most horrifying story I have ever read. vEDS had taken away almost a whole family. Not just one member, but five members of the same family. Yes five people. Aged 48, 40, 42, 49 and 23 years. Not only this, but children. So many children gone way before their time. What else does that? What is there that is so cold that it can destroy a whole family in the blink of an eye? Yet nobody knows about vEDS? Sure it's rare, but it's very real.

As I learned more and more about these people that had been taken away from us, the guilt would only grow. My mother, she hadn't got it, but she was feeling the effects. A lifetime of being by my father's side and now she also had myself and my sister to worry about. All the stress and worry I had brought to her doorstep. The realisation of what I had done was bearing down on me. Strangling me. Sometimes I couldn't breathe. I was beginning to drift away from my family. Hiding from them, knowing that I had brought nothing but pain, heartache and fear into their lives. My mind was beginning to slip slowly away into a dark, dark place. I would continue searching, trying to find something to cling on to, but I was failing. I couldn't find anything to shed a little light, or hope onto the situation.

As Christmas drew nearer I received some more news. The DNA kit that hadn't yet arrived would never be arriving. It was over. No more research. Funding had been cut. That last glimmer of hope to be able to perhaps do something had gone out of the window. I can only imagine that some pharmaceutical company somewhere had decided it wasn't worthy enough of it's grant, because there weren't enough people out there with this to make them money. This wasn't some common disease that they would rake in the millions from creating a miracle cure. Inside me the distant glow had gone. I was becoming consumed with guilt, fear and pain. Encasing me in its thick fog not knowing which way to turn. I couldn't save anyone, I couldn't help anyone. I was useless.

My brother came over for Christmas that year. I hadn't seen him since before being diagnosed. It was refreshing to see him. But it also added to my feelings of guilt. Nothing seemed the same any more, on the outside all I thought I saw were fake smiles. I was convincing myself that they now all hated me. I felt like an outsider that shouldn't be around them any more. Anxiety started to kick in. Sometimes my heart would begin to beat, trying to rip itself out of my chest. Pounding so hard I could feel it shaking my core. My thoughts would begin to fly at me all at once, racing around my head sending me dizzy, making me sick. I couldn't breathe. I was no longer in control of myself, of the situation. I couldn't help them. No one could help them. I couldn't be with them. It was my fault, it was all my fault. I would hide away, under my covers in my bed. Far away from them and far away from the world. My mind was lost. I was no longer the strong willed person I once was.

So a new phase of DABDA then. Depression. A dark lonely place, the prison cell of the mind. My own thoughts driving me mad. All logic and hope gone. Just a darkness that in the space of a few weeks had consumed me. Triggered by events that I had held out so much hope for, but they led to nothing. Putting myself back in this place is not easy. I don't want to remember what I was thinking back then. Because I wasn't thinking straight. Sure, I tried to fight it, tried to pull myself out of the void, but I no longer had any control. There was no sense to be made out of the situation. All I saw was the fear. All I saw was the pain, and the guilt. Amplified by the state of my mind. The positive strong willed guy had left, and what remained was a wreck. A mangled mess of a man with nowhere to turn.

On the final night of my brother's visit it happened. I had been around my parents house where Charlie was staying. I was trying to hide everything that I was feeling away from them. I didn't want them to see what was eating away at me, and I wouldn't let them see. They had enough to contend with. In but a few hours my brother would be leaving to go home. It was late at night and he would be setting off to go down south where he would catch the ferry and drive the rest of the way back to

Germany. I hugged him, said my goodbyes and went home.

Upon returning home I made myself a cup of tea and sat at my computer desk, My black gloss computer desk complete with shiny lights. It took pride of place in my kitchen-cum-games room. I just sat there. No lights on, next to my computer with a cup of steaming tea beside me. I thought of nothing. Just staring at the wall through the darkness, not looking at anything, just a complete blankness. My tea was going cold, but still I sat there, silent, not moving, not thinking. To this day I don't know what exactly happened and why it happened, I couldn't explain it then, and I couldn't explain it now, but it just happened.

Suddenly my eyes begin fill with tears. I could feel them running down my face, over my cheeks and down to my lips, leaving their salty taste. But I still sat there as they began to really stream down my face, nose beginning to run but, motionless, silent and then in one swift motion:

"Aaaaaaaarrrrrrrrrrrgggggggggghhhhhhhhh"

I screamed out loud like some sort of crazed war cry as I ran into battle. I rose up from my stillness, flinging my chair back across the room causing it to crash hard into the wall whilst my right hand swooped through the air. Grabbing my cold tea in one swift motion, I raised it above my head, the contents spilling out all over, and as hard as I could, I threw it across the room in pure rage. As it hit the wall it smashed completely sending fragments flying down to the floor everywhere. Before it had hit the wall I had managed to stomp across the kitchen and found myself yanking out the draw full of utensils, feverishly fumbling around, grabbing handfuls of utensils and sending them flying out behind me until I found what I was looking for.

My hand grabbed round the shaft of a ten-inch sharp

kitchen knife. For a moment I stopped and looked at it. Twisting round I walked towards the chair that I had flipped back across the room, picked it up and seated myself once again.

With knife in hand, I pulled up my left sleeve, passed the knife into my right hand and brought its blade to the top of my wrist. I pressed it down against the skin slightly, then pulled it back sharply towards my body. A sharp sting gave way to the redness, then again, I moved the knife in position and pulled back violently cutting through myself.

Blood began to pour down my arm.

I hadn't cut deep, but I cut enough. As the blood reached the end of my arm it dripped over my knuckles, down my fingertips and dropped onto the floor. I put the knife against my arm and cut again, then again and again.

Blood dripped from me.

I just sat there again, in silence. My arm was stinging. I hadn't cut deep but the blood thinners meant that the blood was running fast. This wasn't me, but it felt good, I felt like I was in control, I made myself bleed.

vEDS wasn't in control of my destiny, I was! Here and now I had complete control of what was happening, I had the power to stop it in its tracks.

I turned my bloody arm over, exposing my wrist, then I raised my knife bringing the point to rest against my wrist. All those infected veins under my skin, weak, broken. I pressed the knife against them not quite hard enough to break the skin but hard enough to feel it, hard enough to let them know that I was now in control of my destiny. I was choosing how it would end, I had the power of life and death, not it, not vEDS. I am the master of my own life and I will not be defeated. You don't own me, you don't control me, I control you. You can fight me but I promise you that you will not win. I am stronger than you can ever imagine possible. You will not silence me!

To this day I don't know why I did it. It was madness. A crazy thing to do, dangerous given the circumstances, but I did it and I have told you. All I can think is maybe that it some way it was my way of getting out of the hole I was being buried in. All that guilt and anger had built up in me and was taking over my life. I wanted to take it back. There was no sense or logic involved but I wanted my mind back, I wanted myself back. These were extreme circumstances under extreme conditions. I had no intention of taking my own life, far from it. Perhaps I was just accepting it in my own way, I really don't know.

On the Monday morning I made an appointment to see my local GP. The events of what had happened over this weekend scared me. What had grown inside of me, I feared its power and admitted that I needed a little help. After all these were life changing events and there wasn't really any help offered. With the little sanity that was left inside of me, I had to seek out my own help once again. I wouldn't let the feelings of guilt take over me and turn me into some kind of monster. My mind cannot recall all that happened, the events seem a little hazy, but I will try and tell you what I do remember.

By some miracle I was able to get in to see a doctor straight away. I had taken my mother with me, as I wanted her to hear what I had done. I couldn't really find a way of telling her one to one, as I felt ashamed, but if I could explain it to the doctor with her there, then she would understand in some way and wouldn't think any less of me. As I spoke to the doctor about the events of the night he seemed a little shocked. I told him of how over the course of a few weeks there was something building up inside. I told him of how my chest would begin to flutter, then my head would begin to spin with horrible thoughts. Thoughts of wanting to flee far away from everyone. I told him of how I struggled to be around my family. The guilt that had built inside of me, overwhelming my every attempt to rationalise, and then of how I had cut myself time and time again. I do remember of how he looked at me with sorrowful eyes and apologised for what happened. Why did he apologise? I'm not sure, perhaps in reality at the time of diagnosis we should have been offered proper emotional support. Perhaps then this wouldn't have happened and it could have been worked through without coming to a head like this. Whatever the reason was, it happened and had to be dealt with. With the fact that I had harmed myself he was obliged to ring the Crisis Team. He told me that they would ring me and come out to visit me at home to talk about these feelings, to help me work through the problems that we now faced, and to check that I was in a safe mental state.

After a few hours of arriving back home I sat around in the empty flat. It was cold, it was silent until the telephone came to life.

"Hello."

"Hi, is that David?" came a soft voice from the other end.

"Yes, yes it is."

"Hello David. This is Michelle from the Crisis Team. We have had a phone call from your doctor and would like to come out and see you if that's alright? How are you feeling?"

"Yeah I'm okay thanks. That's fine, when would you like to come?"

"I'm not far from you at the minute, I can be around in about an hour then we can have a little chat if you would like?"

"Yeah sure, fine."

With that the phone went dead and I sat in silence just waiting.

As this Michelle had said, within an hour there was a knock at the door. The woman in the white coat was coming to take me away, coming to decide if indeed I had completely lost the plot. Of course in reality how can you lose the plot if you never had it in the first place!

Upon opening the door I was very surprised at what I saw. Standing there in front of me was not what I expected. But actually what had I expected? Lately my expectations had become very little, perhaps I was hoping for some wise old woman to come and show me the way, to take my hand and make everything all right again. In reality stood before me was this young lady, she must have only been in her early twenties, she seemed very young to be able to delve deep into my mind and turn back on the light that the darkness had consumed. But as they say, never judge a book by it's cover. I'm sure she had all the relevant qualifications to enable her to help me. Maybe I was just coming to realise that I might just be a little older than I remember myself being.

"Hello David, I'm Michelle, we spoke on the phone, can I come in?"

"Yes of course come in. You will have to excuse the mess a little." Actually it wasn't too messy, I was a regular fan of the hoover and tidying up even though I am of the male variety.

"Would you like a cup of tea or coffee or anything?"

"No, I'm okay thanks, I've had a few too many cups today already."

"Okay. Well follow me then," with that I led her into the front room and we took a seat.

"So David, how are you feeling? I've had a little background information about you. You have been diagnosed recently with a rare syndrome haven't you?"

"Yes I have."

"Would you like to tell me about it? Nice place you have here by the way," Michelle said as her eyes looked around the room.

"Thanks, its not too bad."

I then went into a run down of the events that had happened over the past year leading to the diagnosis of vEDS, I explained what it was and showed her the medical emergency leaflet to give her a better idea. This leaflet was proving a handy little bit of information to explain the basics.

"Blimey" came her reply, "That's quite something."

"Yeah its not the best of things."

"So the doctor tells me you have been struggling a little. Would you like to tell me why?"

Of course I thought the answer to that was pretty simple, but maybe it wasn't so simple.

"Well, it's not really that I'm bothered about myself. The problem is it's not only me that it affects. If that was the case then it would be okay, I could handle that, but there is so much more to it."

"Like what?"

"My sister and my father have also been diagnosed. My father has had problems before, but my sister is a little different, she has had problems but nothing to warrant being diagnosed with something like this. And my mother, my mother has had to deal with so much over the years and now I have brought them this. I have put this on them .."

"But you didn't create this David. From what I know it was already there." Michelle looked me in the eye closely to get my attention.

"I know I didn't, but I found it. If I hadn't found it then we would never have known. We could have just gone about our lives as normal without having to worry about this damn evil thing. I was so insistent on getting to the bottom of it that all I have done is inject terror into our lives. Fear of what's going to happen, pain. No-one can help us, no-one, there isn't a damn thing anyone can do. All I have done is made us all aware we are a ticking time bomb waiting to go off and there isn't anybody out there that can stop it. My mother, my poor mother, she has stood by my father all these years and now, now she has to go through more .."

"You can't think like that though David."

"But I do, and I can."

"Surely it's better to know? They can help you, monitor you and if anything arises then they are in a better position to help you as they know what they are dealing with. But really you shouldn't think like that, anyone could get run over by a bus walking across the street .."

I cut her off here. "Maybe so, but crossing the street you can control, you can do something about it by crossing the street properly. This you can't do anything, you could lie in your bed all nice and safe and then all of sudden you're not so safe."

At this point I may have risen my voice slightly to try and make her understand.

"I know, it must be hard .."

How could she know? Did she have vEDS? Could she contemplate exactly what this was? Did she even know what vEDS really was?

"But you really shouldn't feel like that, you have to look on the positive side of things."

Of course I always did think on the positive side, my glass was always full even when it was half full. The conversation really wasn't helping, in fact it was just making me feel frustrated. Yes she was only trying to do her job, which I am sure she was probably really good at, but I could see this was going to be my fight. This Michelle was trying to hold out her hand and lead me to the proverbial light, but the battle inside my head was going to have to be my battle. The conversation went on for a while longer, I think until she had decided that I wasn't a danger to myself. We discussed the night where I had flung the cup against the wall and grabbed the knife. I told her that this wouldn't be happening again and how I really had no intention of doing anything as silly as that. Whilst my mind was in a dark place I wasn't about to give up on the fight that was laid out before me. As I had told vEDS that night, as if it were a person standing before me, I was stronger than it, and would not give in easily.

Michelle eventually left me to my own devices and over the course of the next week they would be paying regular visits to see how I was doing and making sure I was alright. This visit hadn't left me full of some sort of magical enthusiasm that everything was going to be okay, but it had made me realise that I needed to give myself a kick up the ass. Of course this wasn't going to be easy.

The following week was hard. It was as if vEDS was fighting back against me. There seemed to be some sort of internal battle going on. I had declared war on this thing inside of me, and it wasn't going to take it lying down. It began to attack me, rapidly, taking away my vision. The blotches of light floating around in my eyesight would come at me relentlessly, attacking in waves three to four times a day. Then the pain in the right side of the head, the elephants stampeding through, gaining strength with each new wave of attack. My bed was beginning to become my jail. But during this time my mind was working out a way to counter whatever the evilness was trying to do. I was dispensing the guilt, there was no need for it. I had nothing to be guilty about, for I hadn't brought vEDS upon us. It was already inside of us. It was already lurking in the shadows, waiting for its moment to strike. Remember it had already taken lives in our family before, but I had given us the power to be able to face the enemy, I had taken off its mask so that we could stand toe to toe. This was how we could fight it, by being ready, by being knowledgeable. Knowing what this monster was and what it could do would come to help keep us alive! We would stand tall with countless others from all across the world. Sharing our power and keeping the battle alive everyday.

"Know thine enemy"

During this week, between the countless attacks of visual nightmares, I began to read. A passion that I had long forgotten. As a teenager I loved reading. Many hours were spent shifting through novels by Stephen King, "The Stand" and "Salems Lot". Also Dean Koontz "Sole Survivor", "Servants Of Twilight", to name but a few. Two of my favourite authors filling my mind with tales of the unimaginable, whilst playing 80's and 90's rock ballads in the background. As I read through Stephen King's "Doctor Sleep", I was reigniting what I had once lost. My imagination was being fuelled by the words that were sitting on the pages. My thoughts were turning from the darkness that was keeping me prisoner.

Every waking moment I would read more and more, and within a few days I had finished the book. In turn this brought about a new idea. We couldn't be helped right now, but I was beginning to think of a new way that I could fight back. I knew what I had to do, it was becoming clear. Everything I had gone through in the past had to be written down, to make sense of it all. So I began to write. I sat in front of my computer and the words began to flow from my brain down to my fingertips. I was writing, writing of the events that had happened leading to this day.

The more I tapped away at the keyboard the more I

could start to see the light. The dark inside was subsiding, I was slowly letting go of all the guilt and frustration that had been built up and starting to make sense of all the madness. Suddenly, I had a new purpose and was accepting. Was this the final stage of DABDA? Was this my acceptance? I don't know, but it was helping. I was learning to help myself mentally to deal with the situation at hand, but little did I know that the more I typed, it was giving birth to something else. This new tool was starting to serve another purpose. It was becoming less about me and more about helping. With sheer determination it would be finished.

Slowly but surely the migraines began to die down, and the bouts of vision loss began to dissipate. If this was some sort of revenge attack then I was fending it off and beating it back.

My mind had started to become clearer, the writing really did help. I guess it was some sort of self therapy, making my mind focus and begin to see sense again. As the days went by the guilt lifted and I saw it in yet another light. Knowing about Vascular Ehlers-Danlos was a good thing. It would help us to overcome. It would help us to keep safe. From out of this darkness that had visited me I had found new strength, new goals and would learn to live again. Not only that, my life had taken on a new purpose.

In signing up for the research that I had done with Gwen, I had wanted to do something, anything, and even though the research wasn't going ahead, I realised that I could still have the potential to help people. Even if it was just to make a difference in one person's life, the possibility was still there. And there it was, that tiny flicker of hope beginning to grow again. It was time to move on up and take the fight to vEDS.

CHAPTER 6
NEW BEGINNINGS

Now it was time to deal with the situation at hand, and changes would need to be made. As previously stated I was working in the tyre industry. I was very much in a sales role, however I was also fitting tyres in the depot. This was taking its toll on my body. It had been for years, but now it was all too much. The physical side of the job was beginning to cripple me. I would come home at night and would hardly have the energy to get up the stairs into my flat. I would ache so much that I couldn't sleep. Every bone, every joint and every muscle were being punished, and not only that, what I was doing was dangerous. With every tight wheel nut I was putting all my power into breaking off, I was risking my life.

At any one moment in time that I was putting stress on my vascular system, I was risking another tear on an artery which had the potential to be fatal. Gwen Patroni was right when she protested this was "crazy". Okay, so I may be slightly crazy, in a cool way obviously, but I'm not completely bonkers and I knew this was one of the main things that had to change.

When I returned to work after my short period away I called a meeting with our HR guys. They already knew the situation, although they didn't really know the full details. They knew it wasn't great but they didn't understand just how dangerous what I was doing could be, and in order for me to preserve life I had to tell them and see if there was anything else that could be done. This didn't come without its worries. For years and years I had been doing this, would they understand? Would they have a job for me? I didn't know. The thought of having to leave scared me a little. It seemed like I had possibly become unemployable. Another problem with being diagnosed with a life threatening random condition. If you really think about it, who on earth would want to employ someone that has to potentially take a lot of time off due to complications? Maybe nothing would happen, but there is always that risk and there were always the bad days where you would have no choice but stay in bed all day. I know there are laws in place that prevent discrimination against disabilities but this was different. There is nothing ordinary about vEDS! Personally I didn't want to imagine a life without work.

After a couple of days, the HR manager came to see me. Michael was his name, and a friendly man he was. He would always listen and help you when he could. I was hoping he was going to be able help me.

In the depot we had a small tea room, furnished with a few dirty uncomfortable chairs that had seen many days of oil-stained, dirt-filled overalls sat upon them. Unfortunately in this type of job, being clean was not something you could do. We sat down, had a cuppa and began to chat about the circumstances.

"Right David. How are you doing?"

"I'm not too bad thanks, but obviously we need to talk about the situation."

"Yes, you're quite right. I would have come and seen you sooner, but we know you have been going through it a little, so thought it would be best to leave it a while to give you a little time to decide what you want to do. So this vEDS then? I got that right didn't I?"

"Yep that's the one, Vascular Ehlers-Danlos

Syndrome."

"Tell me more about it? What does it mean exactly?"

"Well as you know, one of my arteries had a tear in it and that's why I was off for those few months. To put it as simply as possible, it is a mutation in the collagen. Collagen is like a glue that sticks us together. In vEDS there is a specific mutation which is mainly to do with the arteries and the hollow organs. It can lead to spontaneous ruptures and any pressure on the vascular system is a big no-no as it can only increase the risks."

As I explained this to Michael I also handed him the emergency medical leaflet that I carried around in my wallet. There was a slight pause whilst he read it.

"Wow. I'm really sorry. I'm not quite sure what to say. You certainly are a rare breed." His face looked a little shocked at the piece of paper that he held in his hand.

"Well we have known that for years even without the vEDS, but it's okay no need to apologise!" I raised a little smile to lighten the atmosphere.

"So isn't there anything they can do?"

"No not really. They have put me on a few tablets, but there is no cure really. It's just a case of monitoring and dealing with complications as and when they arise. Whether they will or not is anyone's guess. It's quite random in it's nature and can't really be predicted. We just have to make sure everything is in place if something does happen."

"So really, doing what you are doing now work wise, is not the best of ideas."

"No, it's not good. If I want to give myself a chance to grow old then I can't do this any more. It's putting a big strain on my body as it is, but I'm also risking my life doing it."

"Well, we are going to have to have a think and see if there is anything else you can do."

"Yeah I was thinking maybe about going onto the

delivery side, driving the vans?"

"To be honest I wouldn't really want you doing that. I think we both know you have been in this job too long and have too much to offer, and besides you would be on your own most of the day which I don't think would be too good."

"Hmm. I suppose you could be right there!"

"Yes. How would you feel about travelling to the offices?"

"The offices, well yeah I suppose I could. Its about 45 minutes away from where I live."

"Is that too far?"

"No I think that would be alright. If it means I'm not doing the physical side then it should help and be safer."

"So if we set you up with a desk over there, you could continue your sales role?"

"Yeah I'm more than willing to give it a try!"

"Alright, well let me get this into place then and you can give it a try."

With that, Michael got up and left. This was great news. I had originally been a little apprehensive about the way this would turn out. I had thought that this would be the end of my employment here. But it seems that they didn't want to say goodbye to me just yet. I had been given another chance to work in a safer environment. Things were beginning to look up a little.

2

Where do we go from here? Well if I'm honest things have been a little quiet recently. At the beginning of March 2014, I started my new office job. Quickly I became wrapped up in my new role. The days were long at first due to all the travelling. An extra hour and a half added onto my day from the driving backwards and forwards. I often considered moving closer to the office, but these thoughts were soon dismissed. In the time that I have been here I have grown accustomed to this village's way of life. Its nice, its quiet and suits me very well. My parents are within walking distance down the road which means that I can drop in on them on the way home. I have found myself trying to help them out a little more, and I started feeling okay again about being around them. I knew that if I was nearby, then if anything happened I could be there within minutes. Of course this was also true of myself, I wasn't alone. If I needed them, which I do, then they could also be here within minutes.

As time went by and we catch up to the present I joined Facebook groups here and there. Getting to know so many people in the same situation as myself. The YouTube videos that I had once seen and scared me, the people in them were all real and they were all out there. The mother of the boy who lost his life too young. An amazing and courageous woman who has devoted her life to gaining knowledge and seeking out answers. She was helping so many people and was making a difference in so many people's lives.

In the recent months I have spoken to countless people who are all outstanding and quite remarkable. In great adversity they all stand tall, not just riding the storm but learning to dance in the rain. Each and every one of them has remarkable tales to tell, so brave, so courageous. Banding together like brothers-in-arms, doing battle with the demon everyday. We may be few, but we are far from alone in our efforts to fend off this horrible monster that resides within. This was reinstalling my faith and hope that one day we may find a cure. Or if not a cure, then at least find a way to live our lives without so much fear and uncertainty. Something to take away the everyday pains.

My problems are only the tip of the iceberg. There are many more who face much more severe challenges in everyday life. Unable to walk, unable to stand, unable to eat. So many varying crippling problems, but still they go on. Vascular Ehlers-Danlos may knock us down, but we shall go on. We shall fight with every ounce of strength in our bodies, because that's what we do. That's what we have been doing since the day we were born sometimes without even realising it. We are all warriors in our own right, we fight for our lives everyday, unseen and unheard. There will be a day though when we shall be seen, our numbers will increase and the medical community will recognise our needs. Many will fall in battle, many have fallen already, but for their memories we will continue to rise above. Awareness will be raised and for the generations to come we will strive to seek out the help and the knowledge that we all so deserve. We are not alone.

My father, well he continues to go on. He turned sixty this year. He has defied everything he has ever been told. A miracle, perhaps, I do not know, but he's still here and still going strong. Nothing can beat him down, unstoppable in his journey. The most amazing man I have ever known, my father, the hero. If anyone can inspire hope into the vEDS community then he is the one. Dissections, heart attacks, the constant barrage of effects that vEDS has brought upon him. Being told he wasn't going to make it so many times, but they were all wrong. He proved this and he walks this land with his head held high, fearless.

My sister, vEDS will not stop her. She continues on her path, her quest to walk up mountains. To rise above the land and look down on the valleys below. Sharing stories of her adventures through blogs. So many amazing pictures of the beautiful landscapes that the world has to offer. Her next challenge is to walk up Ben Nevis, a feat of epic proportions in itself, but with vEDS and the injuries suffered from her car crash, this represents something truly outstanding. This challenge I shall be joining her on. On top of that mountain we shall stand united and look back down upon the earth and raise our middle fingers to vEDS. Unstoppable.

Now I know that life is not going to be easy from here on in, it never has been. There will be times where we will all struggle. Our journey is only just beginning and this story is not going to end here. I look around now and my eyes are fully open. Down this road I have learned to appreciate every waking minute. The world is full of beauty, the world is full of remarkable people. For years to come, I strongly believe that we shall carry on with this life-long battle. We don't have Vascular Ehlers-Danlos, Vascular Ehlers-Danlos has us!!

3

With my ever growing need to understand, to learn more, I have signed up for a Bachelors degree with Honours in Health Sciences. This I know will test my brain power to the limits, pushing the boundaries of acquiring knowledge. It starts in October and will take six long years to complete on a part time basis. I truly do not know where this will take me, but it is another step forward. Something to focus on, sink my teeth into and keep on moving ever forward.

Times are changing and as scary as VEDS is, I refuse

to let it control my life any more. I know that I will stumble and I will fall many more times, but I will keep on getting up and dusting myself off. I don't know how long I will live for, but I will hold on to that glimmer of hope that I shall be able to make it to an age like that of my father.

In June of 2015, I joined my sister Franny on the great trek up to the summit of Ben Nevis. This was an achievement that last year I never thought would have been possible. The highest mountain in the whole of the British Isles and we stood on top, looking down on the world. 1344 metres above sea level. In reality we couldn't see a lot, as it was shrouded in clouds. Even in June, the summit was covered in around 8ft of snow.

Climbing to the summit pushed me beyond limits I didn't think were possible. It was perhaps not the safest of tasks to accomplish given the problems with the carotid artery, in fact it hurt like hell. Slowly but surely though, with plenty of stops on the way up to slow down the heart rate. We made it. The way down again was a physical challenge, the pain experienced was incredible. The whole body screamed out, muscles, joints, every inch of the body yearning to stop, but we kept on fighting, because that's what we do. That's what's inside of us. Determination, strength, courage and endurance to see it through.

Now the day before we climbed up Ben Nevis, I would like to tell you a little more about. For it was on this day that my eyes were truly opened to how much beauty there is in the world around us. Despite everything that we have been through over the years, there are moments when all that is pushed to the back of the mind. This day was one of those moments.

After the long drive up to Scotland, we arrived at the camp-site on the Thursday evening. The camp-site resided on the edge of Fort William, sat in the shadow of

Ben Nevis. The skyline around the site was outstanding, surrounded completely by mountains and greenery. I used to spend many days travelling to the Lake District, a little town called Ambleside, on the edge of Lake Windemere. It was a fantastic little town, but this place dwarfed it in comparison. Everything was twice the size. It truly was like standing in a giants playground.

Along with my sister Franny and my brother Charlie, there were a group of people doing the climb with us. A group of remarkable people I might add. Sitting around a camp-fire that night with people I had never met before, in a magical place. It was so refreshing and relaxing to be out in the wilderness. All the woes in the world would just drift away and the present time was all that mattered. However, there was nothing that could prepare me for what I was going to be shown the next day.

On the Friday, our band of merry men and women were taking us to a place called Steall Falls. A short ten minute drive away from the camp-site and we parked up in a small car park. It was located in a small opening surrounded by trees and mountains either side. At the end of the car park was a small walkway which would lead us to a place of pure untouched natural beauty.

For about an hour, to an hour and a half, we followed the walkway. To our left was a steep mountainside, and to the right was a deep gorge with fast running water flowing way down below. As I have gotten a little older I seem to have developed a little sense of not liking heights, and with that in mind it was probably crazy that the next day I would be attempting to climb up to the highest point in the British Isles. But it was a fear I would overcome.

The path was windy and thin, trying my hardest to stay away from the edge and not look down. Luckily there were a lot of trees, so seeing down the side and into the gorge wasn't easy until the tree-line broke a little. The terrain was quite mild, a few rocks to stumble over along the way, but in retrospect it was quite a gentle walk compared to what Ben Nevis would turn out to be.

The weather that day was outstanding. Forget what you hear about it always raining in Scotland. On this day the sun was beating down it's golden rays casting light and great warmth, and it was in fact one of the warmest days. The skies were completely clear and the truest of blues, not a cloud to be seen. We couldn't have asked for anything better.

As we carried on around the twisty path, with sounds of the rushing water echoing in the ravine below us, we came upon a corner. It was at this corner that everything changed. It was on this corner that, when I went round it my jaw would drop and I would stand there in awe of what I saw before me. I think if I hadn't been diagnosed with vEDS, then I would have never have truly appreciated what I was about to see. As remarkable as it would have looked, vEDS has opened my eyes to see things in a completely different light.

Going around that corner, I was stopped completely and utterly in my tracks. Gone was the deep ravine next to us, gone were the trees embracing us in their shadows, but what lay before us was a majestic sight. The enclosed walkway opened out into a wide valley. A valley surrounded by snowcapped mountains everywhere you looked. The path led through the middle of the valley, the flickering reflection of the light from the brightest of suns, shimmering across the clear glacial waters that had now become a wide stream. Far in the distance, just above the greenery of a tree line, a magnificent waterfall flowed fiercely down the side of the mountain. It was beautiful. Breathtaking. It was like entering a scene from Jurassic Park. The only things missing were the dinosaurs, which I could quite imagine being at home in this place. The land that time and technology had forgot. Untouched by the hand of man.

I stood there speechless, my eyes scanning all around. Slowly. Taking in every last detail and carving out the picture to place firmly in my memory. Losing myself in that moment where time did not exist. This was a place of magic and it is moments like these which make memories that last a lifetime.

So there you have it, for now, this is the story of David Malarky. But it is by no means the end. I am full of hope for the future. Now we know what vEDS is, we are empowered to embrace a new life, new experiences and look at the world with our eyes wide open. This my friends, is just a new beginning ...

To be Continued ...

Conclusion

Vascular Ehlers-Danlos Syndrome is a horrible life threatening condition. In the past few months, I have learned of many lives that have been lost, of all ages. With this news it hits home hard how unpredictable it can be. There are times that I wish I hadn't looked into it, times that I wish I could just run away and hide, forget it ever existed. We can't run from what's inside us though. We have to face it, head on, and not let it control us. Acceptance of something like vEDS, I for one, don't think will ever come. Why would you want to accept it? How can you accept something that is so unpredictable and you don't know from one day to the next what's going to happen? The pains that you feel striking fear into your mind, not knowing whether it is going to be something, or nothing.

Although we are all different in the way that vEDS presents itself to us, it is both a physical and psychological battle. But we will keep moving forward, as we have to.

Knowledge is slowly moving forward. More people are being diagnosed. For instance, it is thought by some, that the prevalence once viewed as 1 in 250,000 could now be as much as 1 in 90,000. With more people being diagnosed and more people becoming aware of vEDS, it gives us a greater chance to live longer lives. It gives us a better chance to be able to live safer lives. Maybe even one day we will find a cure and be able to control the major arterial ruptures that it bestows upon us.

There are many positives out there right now. I have heard of a vEDS mouse model being worked on. With that news it can only bring hope. Then there are all the courageous people who work endlessly to spread awareness. We may be few, but our voices are beginning to be heard and hope is being kept alive by so many.

With each rising of the sun, a new day is born unto the world, new life brought upon the land, new hopes and dreams are fulfilled. It is only a matter of time before the sun rises for us. The day will come when we can say Vascular Ehlers-Danlos Syndrome, and those words will be known throughout the world. Stay strong and keep fighting, we are the invisible warriors.

Resources

For more information on Vascular Ehlers-Danlos Syndrome please visit the following sites:

www.annabelleschallenge.org

www.ehlers-danlos.org

www.edstoday.org

www.ehlersdanlosnetwork.org

www.facebook.com/vedsuk

www.facebook.com/annabelleschallenge

Follow The Author:

www.facebook.com/smithauthor

Twitter: @mjsmithbooks

Made in the USA
Monee, IL
07 April 2022

94332939R10121